TESTIMONIALS OF HEALING

Dr. Ryan Bowman is a respected leader in our profession and a beacon of hope for patients who are lost in the healthcare system. These are the patients who have exhausted all therapeutic avenues and have been failed by the traditional approach of healthcare, conventional medicine. His remarkable intellect and passion for healing combine in his latest book to shed light on the path to recovery and attaining optimal health.

What sets Dr. Bowman apart is his ability to simplify the complexities of health and disease and present solutions that resonate as common sense. He has a unique gift for empowering patients to take charge of their well-being, not just by treating symptoms, but by addressing the root causes of failing health. His focus on the gut-brain connection to whole body health is revolutionary and enables life changing results.

Dr. Bowman provides a roadmap to optimal health, defining the logical and actionable steps to take control of your life journey and health destiny. If you're looking for a transformative approach to wellness that goes beyond symptom management, Dr. Bowman's work is a must-read.

Marianne Abate, DC, CACCP

Dr. Ryan Bowman, a respected figure in the field, inspires hope and offers an empowering roadmap to holistic healing. His latest book brilliantly simplifies intricate health matters, putting you in the driver's seat to address root causes. Dr. Bowman's pioneering emphasis on the gut-brain connection unveils a new frontier in achieving positive outcomes in the most difficult cases. If you're on the quest for answers beyond symptom management, Dr. Bowman's work is an absolute essential.

Dr. Ron Bartay, DC

Dr. Ryan Bowman offers hope to patients lost in the healthcare system. This book simplifies health complexities, empowering readers to take control of their well-being by addressing root causes. Dr. Bowman's focus on the gut-brain connection is revolutionary, providing life-changing results. He offers a roadmap to optimal health with common sense, actionable steps.

Joe Mascaro, DC

Dr. Bowman's new book, *Optimal Healing: Common Sense Solutions to Restore Brain and Body*, is a beacon of hope for those facing chronic or degenerative health challenges. Rooted in expertise and fresh perspectives, this book unveils cutting-edge knowledge and innovative treatments. Dr. Bowman provides credible insights, and challenges conventional thinking, paving the way for optimized healing.

Dr Scott Beavers D.C. DACBSP

Hi I'm Nancy. I'm from Iowa City. I initially came because I had severe gastro problem where my mouth was burning. He treated it successfully but while I was being treated I learned that he treated other things too. I was very surprised to hear that he had a program to treat peripheral neuropathy. I've had peripheral neuropathy for 20–22 years. Something like that. Every doctor I've ever seen—even a neurologist—said that there is nothing you can do. You can take a harsh pill like gabapentin that turns you into a zombie but I didn't like that. So I decided "Why not?" I gave his program a try and I am amazed. Really amazed. My feet actually have feeling. I'm not kept awake. Before I go to sleep, I would be kept awake with burning feet and that just does not happen anymore. I just don't know what to say; it was just a big improvement. I was told by conventional medicine that there is no treatment and there is.

Nancy

This was a truly life-changing experience. I was unable to stand or walk more than a few moments without sitting down before falling. I was using a motorized chair for any walking or having to stand for a while (example: in a line). After 3 months of laser, oxygen and pulse wave treatments I am now able to walk normally and stand a long time without balance or leg fatigue as my blood vessels have gotten better and are rebuilding themselves. The result is independence and overall feeling healthy again! I wish I had heard about this earlier.

Loretta

I'm Pat Brockett from Iowa City. I first came to Dr. Bowman for my knees. I received an invitation in the mail for one of his presentations. So I went and I was very interested in what he was saying. He also talked about neuropathy, which is something that I've had for about 20 years, so I thought I'd give it a try. When I first came in I was having a terrible time getting up from a chair due to pain in both knees. I'd have to use all of the strength in my arms to get up. I could hardly go up and down stairs. I was having pain in my knees during sleep that would wake me up. It would hurt me to walk. I was just having a hard time. I've been doing Dr. Bowman's program and my results have been amazing. My knees feel better and they work better. He also started working on my peripheral neuropathy. I'm now able to move my toes and feet again and I was not able to even move them before. I'm starting to get feeling back on my feet and it's really a miracle. I'm just a different person now.

I'm Jefri from Iowa City and I have witnessed Pat's results she is talking about. I'm not somebody who uses the miracle word lightly, but for me it is a miracle to watch how much better she is. She has life back, energy back. I didn't even know about the numbness in her feet until we had the evaluation. The fact that she couldn't feel anything in her feet! I mean he was poking her and nothing. But now it's back!

Pat

He was actually just lying on the couch; I couldn't get him up. I could tell he was just going downhill and I wasn't going to let that happen. So I was researching new ideas of what to do. He had two back surgeries that were not satisfactory so I really don't recommend back surgery. He is, I would say, like 60% better than he was before because I got him walking. We go to the mall now and do some shopping. We could never do that before and he's more willing to do other things. So when the kids come he's willing to get up and get out. Much more active. I got my husband back. I was worried sick , you know. And I could just see the decline. There was no way I was just going to let him go.

Faye and Joe

For years I struggled with anxiety that at times was near crippling. At its worst I decided to take an SSRI and was ok with the idea of taking it for the rest of my life but always hoped to find a solution outside of pharmaceuticals. I first started doing Neurofeedback treatments and within a couple weeks I noticed major changes that I would call life changing. I still felt there was more that could improve and after my aunt was diagnosed with Lewy body dementia I knew I had to do anything I could to protect my brain. I started with my gut and eliminated gluten from my diet. Again, within just a couple weeks I experienced another life changing benefit. I felt a release from the remaining anxiety, a lift in brain fog, and though I hadn't lost any weight, I felt skinny and people were asking if I was losing weight. The only weight I had lost was the weight of inflammation! I am so thankful for the genuine care for my health that Dr. Ryan has and for his willingness to keep looking for answers that I haven't gotten anywhere else!

Theresa P.

Dr. Ryan is the most amazing chiropractor and the seventh one I saw before finally getting help for my vertigo.

He is extremely intuitive and understands more about the nervous system, as it related to my issues, than any of the neurologists I saw when I was seeking help (This includes UIHC and Mayo Clinic).

When I first came in, I was worn out from exhausting my medical options and tired of explaining my story (to get looked at like I was nuts). Dr Ryan was extremely kind and straightforward and never made me feel crazy.

The staff are fantastic, super sweet, and always make me feel welcome.

Janette Frey

I have been to several different chiropractors throughout my life, but Drs. Christine and Ryan Bowman have set themselves light years apart from every other one. What impressed me the most was the intake. Usually, when I've seen chiropractors before, they ask where it hurts and then immediately start adjusting. Maybe they would take an x-ray, but usually not. Dr. Christine took a series of neck and back x-rays, did a simple procedure to see how my body weight was being distributed, and how my ears, shoulders and hips aligned on each side (spoiler alert—they were not and it was startling to see that). She took her time to get all the specifics of my issue. A few days later, Dr. Christine showed me the x-rays and explained them in clear, plain, language. My mind was blown. No one had ever showed me or explained what was happening on the inside of my body in this much detail before.

While what she discovered in my spine is not reversible, she stated that we could slow it down. And I believe her, 100%. I have total confidence that as long as I do my part, their treatment will keep my spine and body as healthy as it can be. Dr. Ryan is absolutely wonderful on the days when he does my adjustments. The staff is simply fantastic and always greets patients when they walk in the door with a smile. The facility is spotless and relaxing. I definitely recommend Bowman Chiropractic to anyone who is looking to team up with people who genuinely care about you as a person.

Joanie Hoefer

OPTIMIZED HEALING

DR. RYAN BOWMAN, D.C.

OPTIMIZED HEALING

COMMON SENSE SOLUTIONS TO RESTORE BRAIN AND BODY

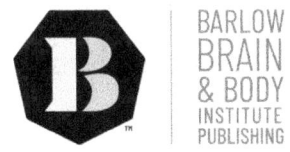

BARLOW
BRAIN
& BODY
INSTITUTE
PUBLISHING

Barlow Brain & Body Institute
266 County Road 506
Shannon, MS 38868
www.barlowbrainandbody.com

I dedicate this to my wife, business partner, and number-one supporter, Dr. Christine Bowman, without whom none of this is possible.

TABLE OF CONTENTS

ACKNOWLEDGMENTS

I would like to acknowledge my parents, Richard and Kathy, in addition to my father- and mother-in-law, Bruce and Jean, for their confidence and support when we began our careers. If you ever doubted our ability to succeed, you never showed it.

FOREWORD

In today's fast-paced world, it is all too common for us to neglect our health and well-being. We often find ourselves caught up in the chaos of everyday life, barely giving our bodies and minds the attention they deserve. However, there is hope. In the midst of this whirlwind, Dr. Ryan Bowman's groundbreaking book, Optimized Healing, offers a guiding light towards a path of true wellness and vitality.

Dr. Bowman's extensive knowledge and experience in the field of healing have allowed him to uncover the fundamental principles that can unlock the body's innate ability to heal itself. In Optimized Healing, he takes us on a transformative journey, showing us how to untangle the intricate web of dysfunction that often stands in the way of our recovery.

What sets this book apart is Dr. Bowman's step-by-step approach, providing practical and actionable guidance that can be implemented by anyone. By addressing key areas such as improving oxygen levels, optimizing glucose levels, stimulating deficient neurological pathways, and addressing autoimmune diseases, he empowers us to take control of our health and make positive changes that can have a profound impact on our well-being.

Furthermore, Dr. Bowman delves into the damaging effects of inflammation, the often-overlooked issue of neurotoxicity, and the importance of gut health. By shedding light on these crucial aspects, he equips us with the knowledge needed to overcome unexplained health problems that may have plagued us for years.

If you or a loved one are currently grappling with a mysterious health issue, Optimized Healing is a must-read. Dr. Bowman's compassionate and insightful guidance will not only provide you with a deeper understanding of your condition but also offer practical solutions that can transform your life. The power to make a difference lies within the pages of this book.

Remember, the right decision can change everything. By embarking on this journey of optimized healing, you are taking a transformative step towards a healthier, happier, and more vibrant life. Let Dr. Ryan Bowman be your trusted guide as you unlock the secrets to optimal well-being.

Wishing you renewed health and vitality,

DR. ANDY BARLOW, DC
Graduate of the Carrick Institute of Functional Neurology
Graduate of the American College of Functional Neurology
Founder of the Barlow Brian and Body Institute

"Let the rest do whatever, while you do whatever it takes."

—GRANT CARDONE

PART ONE

FIRST ORDER PRINCIPLES

CHAPTER 1

WHERE IT ALL STARTED

"The further a society drifts from the truth, the more they will hate those that speak it."

—Selwyn Duke

My story starts in Hutchinson, Kansas, a town of about 40,000…not too urban and not too rural. I had one sister and we got along well; we enjoyed our high school years, though neither one of us were valedictorians or famous hometown sports heroes. We simply enjoyed our regular-sized house near the end of town and the blessings of routine, loving parents, and stability. The unspoken Midwest rules were easy for me to abide by: work hard, use common sense, and when something breaks, figure it out and fix it. Little did I know that these modest beginnings and straight-forward lessons would have such a profound impact on my life, but they certainly have. They've enabled me to solve my own health challenges and find personal and professional success, and I believe they can help others do the same.

Just a couple of years into high school, I hurt my back playing football. I leaned over one day and was unable to stand back up. I stayed in a flexed position, which was very painful. My dad, who has always been a strong advocate of chiropractic, told me to go see his chiropractor. Taking his advice (Midwest rule #4), I called and made an appointment. What I witnessed when I arrived for my first visit caught me off guard, but in a good way. While I sat in this waiting room, I observed the doctor come in, smile, joyfully call out patients' names, and engage with them as they walked down the hallway. The atmosphere and mood was so upbeat, it felt more like a party than a doctor's office. I remember feeling glad I was there and looking forward to the doctor "picking" my clipboard and calling my name. Needless to say, my appointment went well, and I was hooked: someday I wanted to be a fun chiropractor too, and help others feel better.

After high school, I attended community college for a year, then went to University of Kansas, and then to Palmer College of Chiropractic, which was a great fit; I excelled at all of my classes and found them very intriguing. I had found my academic niche. I learned all the parts of the body, the function of each, and how they all worked together. I was taught how to think strategically through health problems. And the job of figuring out natural, common-sense solutions to fix such problems was relatively easy for me. I wasn't opposed to traditional medicine, but chiropractic was holistic in nature and aligned with the principles I lived by my entire life. I loved it! The only "B" I received was in Radiology, a class I took at the same time I met and started dating my wife; I joke and tell my daughter and son—currently in high school—that it was her fault. I've been happily married to my wife, who is also a chiropractor, for almost 25 years now, so it was more than worth it.

Christine and I graduated from Palmer College of Chiropractic in June of 1999, married a week later, and moved to Iowa City. Three months later, we bought a practice and have put our noses to the grindstone ever since, co-managing a clinic that has surpassed our wildest dreams. Working hard—a lesson I learned young—continues to be the main ingredient of our success.

CHAPTER 2

THE STANDARD AMERICAN DIET

"You'll never change your life until you change something you do daily. The secret to success is found in your daily routine."

—John Maxwell

WINNING THE WRONG GAME

Have you ever heard of the standard American diet (SAD)? It's fitting this phrase carries the acronym SAD because that's literally how it makes millions of Americans feel. To truly understand the genesis of the SAD, let's think back a few generations and consider the food our ancestors ate. Most of our grandparents consumed things that grew in the ground, on a tree, or that they killed. They ate real, unprocessed foods, fruits and vegetables, meat that they raised or hunted, eggs from chickens in their backyard, and healthy fats like butter and lard. If they ate bread, it was made at home from flour that was not milled from hybridized, pesticide-laced wheat. In short, they ate real, unmodified, unprocessed food. Now let's compare the diet of our ancestors with the diet of most twenty-first-century Americans.

Today, convenience is king. Fast food rules. Most food comes packaged in a bag, box, or plastic wrapper. Very few people grow their own vegetables and fruit and even fewer raise their own meat. It's easier than ever to buy Wonder Bread, Pop Tarts, or potato chips at the supermarket. The majority of meat animals are raised on commercial farms and fed a diet of GMO corn, soy, and wheat. Eggs are produced in huge factory farms where the hens are fed—you guessed it—GMO corn, soy, and hybridized wheat.

Let's take a look at what a regular, American child eats on the SAD:

> SAD breakfast: low nutritional value pastries, sugary cereal, and milk or orange juice.
>
> SAD lunch: low nutritional value processed food because it's cheap at school.
>
> SAD dinner: low nutritional value sandwich, potato chips, and soda.

The average adult's diet is no different, consisting of fast food, processed food (comes in a bag or box), and soda or, even worse, diet soda. The scarier news is gluten is laced into nearly all of this processed food. Today's food lacks the vitamins, minerals, and nutritional value of the food of our ancestors' era. It's higher in calories, lower in nutrition, and full of more inflammatory factors than ever before. If you don't believe me, look at pictures of the average American family from the 1970s and 1980s. Maybe one person was overweight. Today, one person is likely trim and fit, and everyone else in the picture is fat, overweight, or morbidly obese. We've traded nutrition for convenience, real food for genetically modified and/or hybridized replacements, and quality for quantity. The worst part is people don't understand what they're doing wrong because they've done it wrong for so long that wrong has become "normal." So what's the result of this diabolical diet change in America?

There are three major issues stemming from the low-quality, high caloric nature of SAD. We'll look at each of them briefly in this chapter and then explore in-depth solutions to these problems in subsequent chapters.

PROBLEM #1: GLUTEN SENSITIVITY

Gluten, a protein composite found in wheat, exists in nearly every kind of processed food available at fast food restaurants and on grocery shelves today. The reason modern-day gluten is a problem for our guts (digestive systems) is that modern wheat has been hybridized (Different varieties of wheat have been cross-bred to produce new, modern varieties.) to increase harvest yields and maximize resistance to pests and disease. Unfortunately, our bodies don't have the right enzymes to digest these new varieties. When we eat gluten, undigested protein leaks into the bloodstream where our bodies recognize it as a foreign invader, cueing up our immune system to attack and kill it. This process is like sandpaper rubbing on the gut barrier, similar to a leak in your roof. It starts small but has huge long-term effects. This inflammatory reaction happens every time an "invasion" happens, which for Americans eating the SAD is at least three times per day. Imagine if a robber broke into your home three times per day. You would eventually get tired of fighting off the invader, right? That's what happens to our immune system too. Our body gets tired of fighting and gives up, resulting in autoimmune conditions, fatigue, brain fog, insomnia, depression, anxiety, chronic pain, and so on.

Gluten sensitivity is an exaggerated immune response to gluten that leads to an inflammatory reaction throughout the brain, gut, and body and can lead to an autoimmune response, thereby, causing the immune system to attack, break down, and eventually destroy the brain, gut, and body tissue. The literature recognizes it as a trigger in cognitive impairment, dementia, psychiatric disorders (e.g., anxiety, depression, bipolar disorders, obsessive-compulsive disorders, autism), movement disorders, general neurological impairment, ataxia (lack of muscle control and coordination), restless leg syndrome, neuropathy (numbness, tingling, pins and needles in hands and/or feet), myoclonus (sudden, brief involuntary twitching or jerking of a muscle or group of muscles), myopathy (muscle weakness), multiple sclerosis, cerebellum disease (responsible for controlling gait and muscle coordination), neuromuscular disease (the most common sign of these diseases is muscle weakness), and migraine headaches. As you can see, gluten sensitivity can negatively impact almost everything regarding the nervous system as well as your thyroid gland, joints, and skin.

PROBLEM #2: INFLAMMATORY PROCESSES

Think of inflammation as a fire in your body. If you had a fire in your house, you would put that fire out completely before repairing the damage. This is similar to how inflammation affects the body. It's important to note that not all inflammation is bad. In fact, it serves a great purpose for acute injuries like a sprained ankle. If you twist your ankle playing basketball, inflammation draws the healing processes to the area and starts repairing the damage. However, chronic inflammation is not good. Chronic inflammation, which can be triggered by a variety of dietary or environmental factors (especially the SAD), acts as a river of hot, molten lava going through your body. It's destructive, creates all sorts of secondary problems, and must be eliminated before the body can begin to heal itself.

If you're curious about your body's level of chronic inflammation, here are three of the best indicators. These markers can easily be identified through blood work; however, they will likely not be on the blood panels ordered by your general practitioner. You will need to specifically ask for these markers to be tested.

1) A1C: This should be below 5.6. Levels above 5.6 indicate pre-diabetes and major inflammation.
2) C-Reactive Protein (CRP): This should be below 3 mg/L.
3) Homocysteine: This should be between 5–7 mmol/L.

Let's look at how chronic inflammation manifests in different areas of the body.

1. Body: This causes the tissue destruction of muscles, joints, and ligaments, which leads to chronic pain.
2. Brain: This triggers anxiety, depression, insomnia, and lack of focus and attention.
3. Gut: This manifests as gastroesophageal reflux disease (GERD), irritable bowel syndrome (IBS), bloating, distention, malabsorption disorder, leaky gut, and more.

There's not an exact way of predicting how inflammation will affect each person, but we know it attacks the weakest area of the body first. An invading army doesn't start at the thickest part of the city wall. No, they aim for the wooden gate because it's the weakest spot. The same is true of inflammation. It finds the weakest area of your body and settles there first.

PROBLEM #3: BLOOD SUGAR DYSREGULATION

The SAD is high in sugar and carbohydrates, and consumption of these sugary, highly processed foods drives up blood sugar levels. This poor diet carries a one-two punch: a) inflammation and b) diabetes. Blood sugar or glucose comes from the food you eat and is your body's main source of energy. Your blood carries glucose to all of your body's cells to be converted to energy, but too much sugar in the blood can have disastrous effects. A range of 85–99 mg/dL is considered optimal. Blood glucose from 100–125 mg/dL is considered insulin resistant (the precursor to diabetes), and anything over 126 mg/dL is officially Type 2 diabetes. The higher your blood sugar levels are, the higher your inflammation levels. These two markers go hand-in-hand. Processed food containing gluten combined with a high-carb diet creates an inflammatory cascade that drives up blood sugar and triggers inflammatory processes in the body. This ultimately causes long-term damage to the brain, body, and gut.

As you can see, diet is incredibly important to one's overall health. One of my favorite sayings is, "Man's food kills, and God's food heals." The sad part is that most people have no idea how crucial their diet is to achieving vibrant health and long-term wellness. Why? If a lie is told long enough, people start to believe it. Many of us were never taught that gluten-containing, carb-laden processed foods are bad for us. It's normal, it's the way we were raised, and most everyone is doing it. Yet the research is devastatingly clear: the SAD is destroying our bodies and our health. We can't fulfill our God-given potential if we're slowly killing ourselves with these foods. If you're having chronic health problems but not addressing your diet, it's like having a giant hole in the roof and only worrying about emptying the buckets of water on the floor. To make things better, you first have to stop making them worse.

TWO SCHOOLS OF THOUGHT

When it comes to treating chronic health problems, two schools of thought rule the day.

1. The gut and the brain are completely separate from each other and the rest of the body, therefore, treat them separately.
2. The gut and the brain are interconnected through the vagus nerve, therefore acknowledge the latest scientific research confirming this and treat them together.

Before I knew better, I belonged to the first camp. Now that both I've learned the truth and the scientific research is clear, I've strongly staked my flag in the second one. The brain, body, and gut make up a whole, complete system that works together. If we want to improve chronic health issues like pain or autoimmune conditions, we must treat these parts of the whole simultaneously.

Through working with patients at my clinic, spending hundreds of hours reading the latest medical journals, and walking my personal journey of healing, I've realized three fundamental truths that explain why diet is so critical to health:

1. Gluten is the most toxic food product you can put in your body.

2. Today's processed food lacks the total essential vitamins and minerals that our bodies need to function optimally. The SAD has minimal, if any, nutritional value, and consequently, the majority of Americans are walking around with serious vitamin and mineral deficiencies.

3. What you put in your mouth is either going to heal you or kill you.

I state these truths so confidently because I've tested hundreds of patients at my clinic and reviewed the test results myself. There are three main metabolic tests I use to understand where the cascade of inflammation is originating.

These tests reveal three crucial things:

1. Whether the patient carries the gene(s) for gluten sensitivity or celiac, known as the HLA-DQB1 gene;

2. Whether they have a leaky gut; and

3. Whether they have any underlying autoimmune conditions lurking beneath the surface, and if so, which area of the body has been negatively affected.

When it comes to gluten sensitivity genes, you can carry zero, one, or two of them. If you have none of the genes, it's unlikely for gluten sensitivity to affect you. If you carry one gene, you are less predisposed to having gluten sensitivity than if you carry two genes. Having two gluten genes is the most serious scenario. Out of the hundreds of patients I've tested in my clinic, only two patients have had no genes for gluten sensitivity, and the majority of people carry two. These genes behave like light switches. They can be activated by environmental factors, and, once active, they are very difficult to turn off. It's not surprising that consuming gluten has a high probability of turning them on.

The other problem with gluten is that it's addictive. Why? When it crosses the blood-brain barrier into the brain, it transforms into a gluteomorphin (a morphine like morphine) and docks on your brain's opioid receptor site, known as the nucleus accumbens. You read it right; once gluten enters your brain, your brain receives it as an addictive substance and produces essentially the same response as if you ingested heroin or morphine.

SETTING YOURSELF FREE

By this point in the book, you may be thinking, "Dr. Bowman, how can this all be true? How are my morning toast and cereal the root cause of my acid reflux and chronic pain?" Do you remember what I said earlier in the chapter? Just because we've been told a lie for a long time doesn't make it true. Whole-wheat cereal is not good for you. Sugary cakes and pastries are not harmless treats. Fast food isn't a more convenient way to eat dinner. Just because everyone else is doing it doesn't make it any less harmful to us. Look at your coworkers, church members, and family. Are they healthy or overweight? Full of energy or constantly fatigued? Do they suffer from anxiety, depression, headaches, or insomnia? Just because these problems are common doesn't make them normal. There's a better way to live.

As a friend and doctor, I ask that you please commit to reading the rest of this book. Answers and hope are ahead. We all have an expiration date, so isn't it time to get our acts together? If you're on the fence, think about it this way: you've done it your way up until now, and it's not working. Now, consider an approach that's scientifically proven to work. Start a new chapter in your life today. Your legacy is too valuable to be diminished by chronic health problems. Be responsible to your family; they want to see you vivacious, full of energy, and cognitively healthy too. We can't expect the government, Big Pharma or our insurance companies to fix our issues for us. It's time to commit to your health and vitality.

I ask all my patients, "How far do you want to go?" Now, I'm asking you the same question. How far are you willing to go to reclaim your health?

CHAPTER 3

THE BRAIN-GUT CONNECTION

"I am not a product of my circumstances. I am a product of my decisions."

—Steven Covey

YOUR BREAKTHROUGH UNDERSTANDING

The first step to reclaiming your health is understanding the amazing machine that is your body and how it works. It's not a bunch of individual organs operating independently of each other. Instead, it's an interconnected system working together holistically through constant communication from the brain to the body, the body to the brain, the brain to the gut, and the gut to the brain.

Many of us instinctively understand that our brains and bodies communicate back and forth. For example, you can see a glass of water sitting on the counter and pick it up. Your brain (frontal lobe) sends a signal to your hand, and you pick up the glass. In return, your hand sends a signal back to your brain (parietal lobe) noting the weight, shape, and condensation on the glass. This action is possible because of the brain-body feedback loop. The brain sends a neurological signal to your hand, and in return your hand sends a neurological signal back to your brain. This is the part of the nervous system responsible for executing voluntary actions like picking up a glass or throwing a ball across the yard.

However, there's a whole other part of the system that's easy to forget, the autonomic nervous system. Though we don't often think about it, we're in big trouble if it stops functioning. This ultra-important system controls all of the involuntary actions necessary for living such as our heart beating, lungs breathing, and the subject of this chapter, digestion.

To understand our digestion, we look to one of the main divisions of our autonomic nervous system known as the enteric nervous system, a mesh-like system of neurons that governs the duties of the gastrointestinal tract. We can easily forget about this incredible system because we don't make it function by thinking about it. Instead, the brain and gut talk back and forth on their own about the complex process of digestion.

Many people don't realize that the outside world is what's inside our guts. We ingest food that travels to our stomach, and the stomach sends a signal to the brain saying the food has arrived and it's time to release hydrochloric acid, the substance that breaks down food in the stomach. Next, the broken-down food reaches the small intestine where it encounters epithelial cells. These epithelial cells form a single-layer barrier between what's inside your gut and what gets through that protective lining, which eventually ends up in your bloodstream. Along the way, your brain communicates with your gallbladder, signaling it to contract and release bile. It also talks with the liver and pancreas, perfectly timing the release of critical digestive enzymes that break fats, proteins, and carbohydrates into smaller components your body can easily digest. The small intestine is where your food is broken down, assimilated into your bloodstream, and absorbed, whereas the large intestine's main function is taking water out of your feces before it's eliminated from the body. The large intestine is also home to our microbiome, which we will talk about in a later chapter. As this is all happening, your brain is controlling the speed at which your food moves through your gut, which is known as "gut motility." When the system is healthy, this is all done automatically without our thinking about it.

The main superhighway of communication between the brain and the gut is the vagus nerve, one of the biggest, fattest nerves in the body. The technical term for a nerve like this is "highly myelinated," which simply means it's heavily coated with a thick layer of myelin, basically an insulating layer that forms around nerves. It's made of protein and fatty substances and acts as a conductor for signals sent throughout the nervous system. The more myelinated a nerve is, the faster it can send signals to and from the brain.

You may be thinking, "Dr. Bowman, this information is all well and good, but why does it matter to me that my brain, body, and gut communicate with one another?" To illustrate just how vitally important this topic is to your health, think about your heart. Why is it important that your brain and heart have a healthy, open highway of communication? Because if they don't, your heart stops beating, and you die. Now think about your lungs. Why is it important that your lungs and brain talk back and forth effectively? Same reason, if they don't, you lose oxygen supply and expire within minutes. In fact, a person needs to breathe twenty to sixteen times per minute for optimal function because oxygen is necessary for life. Thanks to the vagus nerve, if you're not breathing as you should, a signal is sent to your brain saying, "Breathe deeply or more often so there's more oxygen supply."

Just as your heart and lung functions are necessary for staying alive, so is your digestion. Your gut health is just as important as your brain health, and the two working in sync are the key to living a healthy, vibrant life. The brain communicates with the gut for the main function of assimilating and breaking down nutrients, and we each need these vital nutrients for our brain to function and our body to heal itself. Like a conductor coordinating the intricate movements of an orchestra, our brain is the grand conductor signaling back and forth with the gut to time these important movements such as secreting hydrochloric acid and enzymatically breaking down fat, protein, and carbohydrates. The way our gut breaks down food, extracts vital nutrients, and gets those nutrients into the bloodstream is what feeds our body and brain, and all of these processes are intricately timed. If even one action happens too soon or too late, the whole process is compromised.

The brain controls and coordinates gut motility and timing mechanisms as each digestive organ signals back to the brain exactly what's happening, ensuring every movement happens on time. The gut and brain constantly communicate back and forth ensuring smooth transitions in motility to successfully break down food for absorption. If this communication fails, malabsorption issues result. Symptoms may include gastric reflux, heartburn, bloating, belching, constipation, and diarrhea. Some of my patients even tell me it feels like a brick is in their stomach.

The brain says what to do and when to do it, and the gut calls back saying, "OK, that's done, and now this is done."

The brain controls the motility (movement of food through the gut), and the gut fires back to the brain saying, "OK, we're at this point of the process. Now we need to get ready for the next step."

Your enteric nervous system (gut) is constantly communicating with your brain saying, "Here's where the food products are, and here's the next step."

Your brain then signals which enzymes are released and how quickly it all must move through the system with the ultimate goal of successful absorption so the body gets the vital nutrients it needs to heal.

We've looked at communication between the brain and the gut; now, let's dig into the ways chronic pain, the brain, and the gut are connected. As mentioned earlier, our frontal lobe controls our movements, like picking up a glass of water. Our parietal lobe receives the sensory input from our hand to feel the weight, shape and condensation on the glass. However, that's only a fraction of the overall function of both the frontal and parietal lobes. The frontal lobe moves the body and controls focus, attention, concentration, goal setting, planning, happiness, overall emotional well-being, social interactions, impulse control, learning, and memory. Our parietal lobe both receives input from the body and helps maintain our balance and awareness of where we are in space. When our frontal lobe is malfunctioning due to chronic inflammation, blood sugar dysregulation, gluten, leaky gut, gut malabsorption issues, and/or autoimmunity, we may start to notice things such as loss of focus, attention, concentration, mental and physical fatigue, anxiety, depression, insomnia, loss of emotional control, lack of social skills, obsessive compulsive disorders, loss of the ability to learn new things, and memory loss. When our parietal lobe malfunctions, we may notice loss of sensation in our feet and hands, loss of balance, cold feet and hands, numbness and tingling in our extremities, and chronic pain syndromes like fibromyalgia. All of these issues are linked to chronic inflammation, blood sugar dysregulation, gluten, leaky gut, gut malabsorption issues, and/or autoimmunity.

The other common source of chronic pain as it relates to the gut starts with the vagus nerve. As I mentioned earlier, this nerve is a superhighway of communication, and when our brain fires a signal down to the enteric nervous system (responsible for communication in the gut), it does so via the vagus nerve. Chronic inflammation, blood sugar dysregulation, gluten, leaky gut, malabsorption issues and/or autoimmune disorders can all slow down or damage the transmission of signals between our brain and gut or body, leading to a multitude of chronic health problems like anxiety, depression, insomnia, chronic pain syndromes, memory issues, balance disorders, gastric reflux, heartburn, bloating, or constipation. But, no worries, your doctor has a prescription for every symptom above (sarcasm intended).

This reminds me of a fifty-six-year-old female who came to my office suffering from mental fatigue, anxiety, insomnia, and chronic pain all over her body. She had almost given up any hope of recovery. During our conversation, I asked about her gut function and past trauma (e.g., car accidents, sports-related injuries). She gave the usual response to gut issues: gastric reflux, constipation, bloating. Her first car accident was at age seventeen, rear impact, and the second at age thirty-five, driver's side impact. (We'll talk more about trauma and its impact on brain-gut health in the next chapter). Her neurological exam revealed cold hands and feet and sensory issues in her feet. All motor reflexes were slow, and her balance was terrible. When she put both feet together, she fell to the right in two seconds. (You should be able to hold that position for fifteen seconds.) These are just a few of the tests I performed to evaluate her frontal and parietal lobe function.

We also completed the metabolic blood work program. She had chronic inflammation, her glucose was high, her liver was not functioning properly, and she had both gluten genes and malabsorption issues. She also had two positive tissues from her Cyrex Array 5 autoimmune test as well as a leaky gut from the Cyrex Array 2. Working to rehabilitate her brain and gut function simultaneously, we began seeing improvements within four weeks. She went from a bummed-out fifty-six-year-old in constant pain to a happy, friendly person full of energy. I share her story to show that by working with your gut and brain, your body can heal and accomplish things you never dreamed it could. Now, let's go deeper into the source of chronic pain and how we treat it.

PART TWO

PAIN, GUT, AND THE BRAIN

CHAPTER 4

THE UNEXPECTED SOURCE OF CHRONIC PAIN

"When you stop chasing the wrong things, you give the right things a chance to catch up."

—Lolly Daskal

THE SECRET SOURCE OF PAIN

W ould you be surprised if I told you the most common source of chronic pain is past trauma? Most people only think of trauma as physical, yet the truth is the brain can't distinguish between physical and psychological trauma. I almost exclusively see patients with a wide array of chronic health problems, and every single one of them has some kind of past trauma from ten to fifteen years prior, and some patients as far back as thirty or forty years. To better understand this concept, let's look at the way physical trauma affects the brain in the long-term.

Car accidents, concussions from sports-related injuries, and traumas from extreme emotional events (known as post-traumatic stress disorder or PTSD) affect the brain in similar ways. The brain is home to a type of cell known as microglial cells. They are found in the central nervous system, and their job is removing damaged neurons, infections, and other debris from the brain and spinal cord. When the brain is damaged by concussion or severe emotional trauma, these cells are turned on. Once they're on, they're very hard to turn off. When they remain chronically on, they begin damaging and destroying healthy brain cells. Studies have shown that chronic blood sugar dysregulation, chronic inflammation, and gluten can also trigger the effect.

When this happens, the frontal cortex is usually affected first. The symptoms manifest as smaller things like focus and attention disorders. If those early symptoms aren't addressed, it progresses into the next stage of anxiety, depression, insomnia, and memory disorders. If those symptoms aren't addressed, the trouble moves to the parietal lobe and manifests as chronic pain disorders.

Psychological trauma works similarly to physical trauma, which is received by the brain as emotional stress, yet the brain doesn't distinguish between physical and psychological stress. Say a woman receives a letter from the IRS: stress. Then she loses her job: stress. A loved one passes: stress. Covid hits home: stress. Stress, stress, and more stress. This psychological trauma will actually affect her physically by changing her brain function and sending stress responses down to the gut, creating problems there as well. Chronic stress is devastating to the brain, particularly the frontal lobe, because it cues the release of excess cortisol, which in turn damages the hippocampus (a complex brain structure embedded deep in the temporal lobe that plays a major role in learning and memory) and leads to memory disorders like Alzheimer's disease.

But wait, how does all of this relate to the root cause of chronic pain? When any aspect of your neurology slows down, the brain tissues get close to threshold, which simply means they fire easily, like having a hair trigger on a gun. Nerves get too close to threshold and require very little stimulation to make them fire, which leads to overactive nerve responses and manifests as chronic pain syndromes like hyperalgesia and allodynia. For someone with either of these conditions, things that shouldn't normally be painful like swiping a cotton ball over the skin or being lightly poked with a toothpick register as intense pain because their nerves fire too easily.

Chronic stress also has a drastic effect on the brain-gut connection. Think about the way people experienced stress ten thousand years ago; they had periods of intense stress, like out-running a saber tooth tiger, and then the stressor disappeared. When a person is in a stressful, life-threatening situation, their body doesn't care about digesting food. It cares about survival. The same principle is true today. Gut motility slows down in times of stress, even chronic stress. Instead of passing through in twenty-four to forty-eight hours, food stays in the body and rots.

Yuck.

Slow digestion creates a cascade of negativity like bacterial and yeast overgrowth, gastric reflux, bloating, constipation, and so on: an entire cascade of dysfunction all because chronic stress slowed the brain down.

In summary, the brain slows down from these five things:

1) Chronic Stress
2) Past Physical or Psychological Trauma
3) Gluten Sensitivity
4) Blood Sugar Dysregulation (via the SAD)
5) Chronic Inflammation

Gluten sensitivity, blood sugar dysregulation, and trauma: what do all of these conditions have in common? They cause chronic inflammation, and chronic inflammation affects the brain, body, and gut. Inflammation of the brain turns on the aforementioned microglial cells, which eventually slows down the brain's function. When brain function slows down, the vagus nerve doesn't fire as well, which leads to gut dysfunction.

I describe patients as a "web of dysfunction" because one, two, or all of these factors could be contributing to their chronic health problems, and very few doctors piece all of these triggers together. This is also why lab work and tests like those at Cyrex and Enterolab are so important. They help me peel back the layers and see what's going on within a patient's body. The cause of chronic pain is often overlooked, and instead of finding the root cause(s), traditional physicians prescribe painkillers or other medications that treat the symptoms rather than fixing the real problem.

THE SEVEN KEYS

1. Oxygen
    One of the big three elements the nervous system needs to function at its peak level, oxygen is necessary and essential for life. Anoxia (which means "without oxygen") equals death. Oxygen is the deal-breaker when it comes to neurological health. The less oxygen we have in our bodies, the more things start to malfunction and the less capacity our bodies have to heal themselves.

2. Glucose
    Second of the big three elements, glucose is your blood sugar. It's the fuel that your body needs to heal itself. It's also needed for the nervous system to self-regulate and function optimally. A good metaphor is that it's like the gasoline for your car engine. Cars run at a certain octane level, and if that level gets out of balance, the car isn't going

to run properly. If our blood sugar is too "low in octane" or too "high in octane," it can't function at its optimal level.

3. Stimulation

    Third of the big three, stimulation's importance can't be overstated. As Einstein once said, "Nothing happens until something moves," and in the body, no healing happens until something is stimulated. Without stimulation, the body's systems weaken and fail. With proper stimulation, those systems thrive and remain strong, which is called neuroplasticity.

    Oxygen > Glucose > Stimulation = Neuroplasticity

4. Autoimmune Disorders

    Autoimmune disorders are kind of like "friendly fire." They develop when our immune system starts attacking the body instead of a foreign invader. Our immune system should only kill the "bad guys" like viruses and bacteria, but when it begins malfunctioning, it doesn't just destroy antigens, it also attacks our own tissues.

5. Chronic Inflammation

    Logic tells you that if your house is on fire, you don't start rebuilding it until after the blazes are put out. Well, inflammation is like a fire in your body, and it can't start to heal until that fire is gone. True healing cannot take place until your body's inflammation is reduced.

6. Neurotoxins

    Neurotoxins are anything that's taken into the body that causes neurological damage. Unfortunately, neurotoxins are much more common than you may imagine. Table sugar is a neurotoxin. High fructose corn syrup is a neurotoxin. The artificial sweetener Aspartame is a neurotoxin.

Drinking water out of a disposable plastic bottle is neuro-toxic. We'll talk more in upcoming chapters about how to eliminate these harmful toxins from your life.

7. Gut Health

It's very simple, 70 percent of your immune system is in your gut. The role of gut health can't be overstated because poor gut health is a trigger for autoimmune conditions and out-of-control inflammatory responses. We must heal our guts to heal our brains and bodies. If you have a bad brain, you're guaranteed to have a bad gut. If you have a bad gut, you will have a bad brain. It works both ways. We must restore optimal gut health and reconnect the gut-brain axis to achieve true healing.

While each of these seven areas is important to address individually, their true power for healing comes alive when we realize that all of these elements are interconnected. Gut health and autoimmune conditions are connected. Neurotoxins and inflammation are linked. Oxygen and stimulation are crucial to one another's roles. The body is a holistic system that must be in homeostasis to heal itself and function optimally. By keeping these seven primary keys in focus, your health can transform from symptom mitigation to a state of true healing and regeneration.

CHAPTER 5

THE VAGUS NERVE

The secret of change is to focus all your energy, not on fighting the old, but on building the new.

—Socrates

THE VAGUS NERVE

We've touched on the vagus nerve in previous chapters, but this incredible "highway to health" easily deserves its own chapter. In the next few pages, we're diving deeply into the purpose and function of the vagus nerve, its relation to our overall health, and a few simple ways we can support this superhighway of communication through positive daily habits. By the conclusion of this chapter, you'll be a vagus nerve aficionado.

Let's begin by defining what the vagus nerve is and what it does. It is one of twelve pairs of cranial nerves, and each of these nerve pairs controls a specific area of the body. Cranial nerve number one deals with smell. Number two deals with vision. Number three controls eye movements and constricts our pupils. Numbers four and six also move our eyes. Number five deals with chewing and sensory functions of our face. Number seven controls the muscles of our facial expressions and salivation. Number eight deals with hearing and balance. Number nine controls salivation. Number ten (the vagus nerve) deals with sensation at the back of the throat, heart rate, breathing, and digestion. Number eleven controls the trapezius muscles, and number twelve controls our tongue.

Here are a few more fun facts about the star of this chapter, the vagus nerve. The Latin word "vagus" literally translates as "wandering." The words "vagrant," "vague," and "vagabond" come from the same root. It's the longest cranial nerve in the body, which is likely how it earned its nickname "the wanderer." Our autonomic nervous system is made up of two parts: the sympathetic and parasympathetic nervous systems. The sympathetic nervous system activates the fight-or-flight response during a threat or perceived danger, and the parasympathetic nervous system restores the body to a state of calm. Cranial nerves three, seven, nine, and ten are all part of our parasympathetic nervous system (aka our "rest and digest" system).

Our sympathetic and parasympathetic nervous systems should be in homeostasis to work optimally. If we're under stress and our sympathetic nervous system gets activated, we're no longer in a rest-and-digest state; we're in a fight-or-flight mode. When we're in this state, salivation and digestion slow down because our body thinks, "Hey if the threat catches me, it doesn't matter if my food is digested or not." These are natural, God-given neurological responses designed for equipping us in immediate, stressful situations. This response should be quick and then dissipate. Unfortunately, in today's society, we're under constant stress, and this sympathetic system is ramped up all the time. The parasympathetic system isn't coming back online, so we're not resting and digesting as we should be.

How does all this chronic stress affect our friend the vagus nerve? Part of its role is maintaining optimal heart rate, breathing, and digestion. When we're under chronic stress, the vagus nerve cannot properly do its job, leading to an increased heart rate or rising blood pressure. Consequently, we begin breathing too rapidly which leads to a build-up of carbon dioxide in our body. If that happens, we can't properly rid our bodies of toxic waste. The vagus nerve is also critical in healthy gut function and controls nearly every step of our digestive process.

Let's walk through the steps of digestion so we can better understand how this system works.

When we take in food and chew it up, that's a voluntary function, but after we swallow, every step of digestion is involuntary, meaning we don't make it happen through conscious thought. As we swallow, the vagus nerve controls our upper esophageal sphincter, basically a valve near the top of our esophagus that makes sure food and liquids go down the right pipe. If this sphincter isn't functioning properly, we swallow air into our stomach, which causes bloating, belching, or gas. Another sign that your valve may be leaky is if you're regularly getting food and liquids down your windpipe. This happens occasionally to everyone, but if it's happening often, it's a symptom that should be noted.

The next step of digestion is the food passing through the lower esophageal sphincter. It's also controlled by the vagus nerve, and if your vagus nerve is not functioning optimally, this sphincter may not close all the way. We have an acidic stomach which should have a pH level of 1.5–2.5 when digesting our food. If our lower esophageal sphincter isn't closing all the way, this stomach acid can back up into our esophagus.

Next, the food enters our stomach. When this happens, the vagus nerve triggers the release of hydrochloric acid (HCL), which breaks down our food into a liquid called "chime." HCL plays an important role in breaking down food, but its presence also triggers a domino effect, cueing several other important steps of digestion. While it's breaking down food in our stomach, it's also designed to kill bacteria, viruses, and parasites that may be in or on our food.

AGE AND THE PRODUCTION OF HCL:

Nearly every one of my patients over the age of sixty doesn't naturally produce enough HCL to support proper digestion. To counteract this aging effect, I suggest using an HCL supplement from Apex Energetics called Enzymix-Pro (K-99). This formula combines a broad spectrum of enzymes to help support the digestion of sugars, starches, fibers, proteins, and fats. It also includes HCl for further digestive support.

If we have problems with our vagus nerve, we'll potentially have issues swallowing, experience gastric reflux, or produce an insufficient amount of HCL to digest protein or kill the bad bugs on our food. The vagus nerve controls all of the functions of our stomach, gallbladder, liver, pancreas, small intestine, and two-thirds of the large intestine. This lengthy "wanderer" controls everything from the "hangy-downy thing" at the back of your throat (uvula) to the upper portion of your colon. Physically, it travels from the back of your throat almost to your belly button.

For successful digestion to happen, every step of the process must be on point, cueing the next function in perfect rhythm just like a row of dominos. For this whole system to work in harmony, the vagus nerve serves as the superhighway of communication between the brain and the digestive system. Every part of the digestive system sends messages back to the brain saying, "Hey, this is what we're doing down here." If these organs start going rogue and acting of their own accord, they get out of sync, malfunction, and food products can't be assimilated properly, which sets up the perfect conditions for a disease process to take root.

The most amazing fact about the vagus nerve is that only 20 percent of its job is sending signals from the brain to the gut. The remaining 80 percent of its function is sending messages up to the brain from the gut. For example, once food reaches the stomach, the stomach sends a message back to the brain saying, "Hey, I'm releasing the right amount of HCL."

The gallbladder says, "Yep, I'm secreting bile."

The small intestine says, "Yes, my tight junctions are closed off so bad stuff doesn't get into the bloodstream."

The large intestine says, "Yep, I'm doing my job and removing water from the stool."

Then the microbiome says, "Yep, I'm assisting in the regulation of the immune system."

All of those messages are sent up through the vagus nerve to the brain to let it know everything is under control down below. Even more amazing is that all of this is happening without our conscious thought. Our conscious mind is completely unaware of this activity until we've damaged enough tissue that we're having pain, bloating, distension, constipation, diarrhea, or gastric reflex. That's when symptoms show up.

Envision digestion as a road trip. The journey has a set route getting you from point A to point B. If the car runs well, you have enough fuel, and you read your map correctly, the road trip goes smoothly and you reach your destination without a problem. However, if you have a flat tire, run out of gas, or miss your turn, the trip becomes complicated in a hurry. Digestion is the same way. If something breaks down from the point where we swallow our food until it reaches our colon, we get symptoms that may lead to disease processes. So, what are the first signs of breakdown? Gastric reflux, bloating, distension, diarrhea, excessive gas, and constipation are some initial signs of dysfunction. If they aren't addressed, these early symptoms progress into disease processes such as inflammatory bowel syndrome (IBS), gastroesophageal reflux disease (GERD), and small intestinal bacterial overgrowth (SIBO).

You may be surprised to hear that conditions like multiple sclerosis (MS), Parkinson's disease, fibromyalgia, ADD, ADHD, and dyslexia are also hugely related to gut function. Nearly every neurological disease starts in the gut before manifesting in the brain, and all of these conditions, if caught early enough, may be helped. The most effective way of healing the body is by addressing all three areas, brain, body, and gut, at the same time. We can make progress by treating the gut exclusively, the brain exclusively, or the vagus nerve exclusively, but true transformation happens when all three are treated simultaneously.

THE NERVE IN ACTION

Think of the vagus nerve as a telephone wire. The brain is on one end of the conversation and the gut is on the other. The vagus nerve is the phone wire enabling communication between the two parties. When the phone system is working well, they speak clearly, quickly, and efficiently, allowing both parties to get their messages across. When the phone line is garbled or has a dead spot, the messages get mixed up. Imagine your spouse calling and asking you to pick up some chicken for dinner. They clearly say "chicken," but just as the words come out of their mouth, you hit a dead spot, and it sounds like "broccoli" instead. You happily pick up broccoli from the store and head home, excitedly giving your spouse their requested ingredient, but alas, it was the wrong thing and dinner is ruined. Communication is important.

In the same way, a healthy vagus nerve ensures clear communication between the brain and gut. An unhealthy vagus nerve isn't just a dead spot of thirty to forty-five seconds, it's a 24/7 malfunction that doesn't correct itself until you see a professional who can diagnose the problem and help you get the system back online.

You may be wondering, "If keeping the vagus nerve healthy is this important, what can I do in my daily life to support it?" Excellent question. Before we get into supporting it, let's talk about what to stop doing. Here are three things you may be doing in your daily life that are unconsciously harming your vagus nerve:

1. Getting on social media (e.g., Facebook, Instagram) or turning on the news first thing in the morning, creating chronic stress. Right out of the gate, this hits your nervous system with bad news, negative thought processes, and comparisons. That inundation with bad news leads to stress. That constant stress causes an imbalance between the sympathetic and parasympathetic nervous systems, which raises our heart rate, slows down digestion, and causes a cascade of other dysfunctions.
2. Eating a SAD. The standard American's morning looks something like this: wake up, gripe and complain about going to work, eat a sugary, carb-laden breakfast (e.g., pastry, pancakes, sugary cereal) chock full of gluten, hydrogenated oils, and other preservatives, then turn on the news

or get on the internet and be inundated with stress. In this morning routine, the body is hit with physical stress (bad diet) and psychological stress (complaining, negative attitude, and bad news). The body doesn't differentiate between those two forms of stress that put an extra load on the vagus nerve, and the inflammatory processes triggered by these foods can damage our brains, nerve function, and gut function.

3. Living a sedentary lifestyle. A sedentary lifestyle is directly hurting your vagus nerve by not stimulating your brain through exercise, and thus not stimulating your vagus nerve. Studies have shown a direct correlation between muscles getting smaller and your brain actually shrinking. Movement is vital to brain health, and brain health is vital to gut health because of the vagus nerve connecting them.

Three things I can do to support my vagus nerve:

1. Exercise: The simplest way to do this is by walking. When you stimulate the body through exercise, you also stimulate the brain, which stimulates the vagus nerve. This has wonderful effects on your gut-brain connection. Make a commitment to move at least four days per week for twenty minutes per day.

2. Deep breathing exercises: This is an ultra-simple way of supporting the vagus nerve. At least once per day, intentionally focus on inhaling for eight seconds, then exhaling for sixteen seconds, ten times in a row. This rush of oxygen stimulates the brain and supports the vagus nerve's function.

3. Ice bath or cold shower: Ice baths or cold showers stimulate our sympathetic and parasympathetic nervous systems, decrease our stress response, improve our immune system, aid in weight loss, and improve tissue recovery processes, all of which contribute to a natural high, boosting mood and attitude. A simple way to start this habit is by incorporating it into your daily shower. Take your normal, warm shower, then turn on the cold water for one minute at the end. Once you're regularly doing this, progress to having the warm water on for two minutes, then cold water for one minute, and do that for three cycles. Note: Please speak to your doctor before starting ice baths.

All of these exercises and habits are grounded in commitment. We all have an expiration date, and we must take action today and every day to ensure our bodies are as healthy as possible. Next let's dig into the ABCs to Health that will give you an initial road map to follow.

CHAPTER 6

THE ABCS TO HEALTH

I believe that the only courage anybody ever needs is the courage to follow your own dream.

—Oprah Winfrey

ABCs TO HEATH

This is one of my favorite chapters because what follows is a simple recipe for drastically improved health: the ABCs TO HEALTH. If you follow these steps, your life and health will be revitalized. Your inflammation will decrease, your body function will increase, and your brain (and vagus nerve) function will increase as well. All of these wonderful benefits come from making small but important lifestyle improvements. Chronic diseases are also known as "lifestyle diseases" because it's often our daily habits and lifestyle that create them over time. In the same way, we can change our habits using the ABCs to Health as our guide and reverse many of the symptoms of chronic disease.

This book is all about the gut-brain-body connection so before we define the ABCs TO HEALTH, let's discuss why they matter to this vital superhighway of communication in our bodies.

1. By following the ABCs TO HEALTH, your overall inflammation will decrease, which lessens the strain on your brain, vagus nerve, and gut and allows your body to heal itself.

2. Your brain health and function will improve, which also supercharges your healing journey.
3. The overall health of your microbiome will improve.

What is your microbiome, you ask? The human microbiome consists of 100 trillion symbiotic microbial cells, primarily bacteria, located in our guts. There are ten times more bacteria, fungi, and viruses in the gut microbiome than cells in our body, and it weighs about three pounds, which is similar to the weight of a human brain. Nevertheless, the gut microbiome has long been forgotten. Only within the last five to ten years has the world of scientific research homed in on understanding this amazing ecosystem inside of us. Rest assured, by following the ABCs TO HEALTH, your gut microbiome will soon be thriving.

Let's dive into this quick action guide for fast-tracking your health. Just as you follow a recipe to bake a cake or make cookies (gluten free, of course), this is the recipe for optimizing your health. If you follow this recipe, good things *will* happen.

ABCs TO HEALTH: THE ACRONYM

A. Antioxidants
    Why They Matter: Antioxidants are our body's defense against free radicals, a type of unstable molecule made during cellular metabolism (the set of chemical reactions that occur in living organisms to maintain life), that can build up in cells and cause a state known as oxidative stress. This may damage your DNA and other important structures in your cells, and this damage can increase the risk of cancer and other diseases. Although free radicals

are produced naturally in the body, lifestyle factors such as trauma, stress, poor diet, or living a sedentary lifestyle can accelerate their production.

Imagine a boxing match where in one corner we have the free radicals, and in the other corner are the antioxidants. Free radicals are the bad guys and antioxidants are the good guys. The bell dings, and the free radicals and antioxidants duke it out. Antioxidants defeat the free radicals by neutralizing them which decreases overall inflammation in the body. Basically, increasing antioxidants means decreasing the harmful effects of free radicals.

Today's Action Step: Increase your consumption of antioxidants by eating more carrots, broccoli, asparagus, berries, artichokes, kale, cabbage, and beets. The natural color of a food is a great indicator of its antioxidant content so make your plate as colorful as naturally possible.

The Next Level: The Next Level: supplement with antioxidants based upon your specific needs.

B.   Brain-Based Therapy
Why It Matters: It's always the right time to take care of your noggin. We need a healthy brain to function in society, and it's also crucial to digestion and gut health because it's the start of the vagus nerve.

Today's Action Step: Get off the couch and get walking. This is the easiest, fastest way of activating and stimulating your brain function, and since stimulation is one of the seven keys to health, the brain must be stimulated to maintain optimal function.

The Next Level: Schedule an appointment for a BrainCore Mind brain map. This is a computerized system that takes a functional image of your brain. It tells us not only which lobes of the brain are weak and need help but also shows in detail which lobes of the brain are healthy and functioning properly. The procedure takes about forty minutes.

C. Clean Gut and Clean Brain
Why It Matters: In the last few decades, poor nutritional habits, stressful lifestyles, and chemical exposures have created significant health problems for our society. We can fight these environmental factors by supporting two of the body's key functions: digestion and detoxification. Detoxing (cleaning out) the brain and the gut simultaneously multiplies the positive effects of detoxification and removes the toxin load hampering our body from doing its number one job, healing itself.

The body's accumulated toxins are embedded in different tissues like fat and connective tissues. Before removing these toxins from the body, they first must be mobilized aka "released" from the areas where they're hiding. After they're mobilized, they enter the detoxification pathways, and after the detoxification reactions, the leftover compounds are excreted from the body.

Today's Action Step: Start supporting your body's digestion and detoxification using something you likely have in your pantry, apple cider vinegar. Make sure it's an unrefined vinegar containing the "mother," which is the healthy, good-for-you bacteria formed during the fermentation of the vinegar. Combine thirty-three ounces of water with two ounces of apple cider vinegar and drink it throughout the day.

The Next Level: Commit to doing Apex Energetics' "Repair & Clear™ Program" a ten-week system specifically designed for powerful detoxification and digestive support.

S.   Stop the SAD Diet and SAL Lifestyle
Why It Matters: As we've discussed in earlier chapters, the SAD is devastating to our health. It is chock full of gluten, unhealthy fats, sugar, excessively starchy carbohydrates, and other inflammation-causing foods. There's zero chance of reclaiming health and vitality if we continue eating this way, and the Standard American Lifestyle (SAL) isn't any better. It's sedentary, lacks physical stimulation and exercise, and relies on hours of TV or other screen time for numbing the negative emotional, physical, and mental side effects it causes. SAD and SAL must go if restoring our health and promoting our bodies' abilities to heal themselves is our goal.

Today's Action Step: Stop eating gluten and processed foods because we can't start getting better until we stop making it worse. Commit to walking (preferably outdoors) for 20 minutes per day, four times per week.

The Next Level: Eat fruits, vegetables, salads, raw nuts (almonds, walnuts, pecans), organic meats (bison, beef, chicken, fish, wild game).

T.   Time Out, Relax, and Reset
Why It Matters: Taking a moment for quiet reflection and relaxation gives your brain the time it needs for a "reset."

Stress is one of the leading causes of inflammation, leaky gut, depression, anxiety, and insomnia. Focusing on deep breathing and meditation encourages your brain to return to a rest-and-digest state, letting your body know it doesn't need to worry about fight-or-flight anymore.

Today's Action Step: Sit in a quiet room and do focused deep breathing exercises for ten minutes. Turn your phone off. Focus on positive things rather than negative things. Think about a loved one or a vacation you want to take. Listen to nature sounds.

The Next Level: Create a daily habit of meditation and focused breathing. Bonus points for doing it twice per day. Get a massage once a month. You deserve it.

O. Omega 3 Fish Oil

Why It Matters: Omega 3 fish oil is a wonderful health supplement for restoring brain and nerve function. Seventy-five percent of the weight of our brain is fat, and the myelin sheath (coating around our nerves) is also made of fat. Fatty fish is a rich source of Omega-3 fatty acids, a major building block of the brain. Omega-3s play a role in sharpening memory and improving mood, as well as protecting your brain against cognitive decline.

Today's Action Step: Take a high-quality Omega 3 supplement every day. If you've had bad experiences with fish oil supplements, you probably weren't taking a high-quality version, or you may have gallbladder issues.

The Next Level: Take a high-quality Omega 3 supplement every day and eat fatty fish like salmon, mackerel, tuna, herring, and sardines two to three times per week.

Nuts and seeds like flaxseed, chia seeds, and walnuts are great sources of Omega 3 as well.

H.   High-Fiber Diet
Why It Matters: Eating a high fiber diet helps regulate the body's use of sugars, helping to keep hunger and blood sugar in check. Fiber also supports regular bowel movements and consistent digestion.

Today's Action Step: The old saying goes, "An apple a day keeps the doctor away," and it's still true. Eat real fruits and vegetables, not fruit juice. Aim to eat one fruit per day and at least one green, leafy vegetable per day.

The Next Level: Drink a daily smoothie containing protein, fat, fiber, and greens. Excellent sources of fiber include chia seeds, whole fruits, and vegetables.

E.   Exercise with Oxygen Therapy (EWOT)
Why It Matters: Forced breathing exercises activate your frontal lobe and increase the oxygen supply in the body. Oxygen is needed to optimize brain and body function.

Today's Action Step: Keep your brain and body strong by walking for at least twenty minutes per day, four times per week. While walking, do forced breathing exercises to supercharge your brain's oxygen supply.

The Next Level: Supplement with nitric balance (K-62) from Apex Energetics. It helps dilate blood vessels for improved circulation, mental clarity, and body performance.

A.   Avoid Gluten and Casein

Why It Matters: Avoid gluten and casein (the protein in dairy) at all costs as they can lead to inflammation, leaky gut, and many other chronic diseases.

Today's Action Step: Remove gluten and dairy from your diet and take GlutenFlam (K52) from Apex Energetics anytime you eat out or may be exposed to cross-contamination of gluten or casein.

The Next Level: Take the Enterolab A2 test, a panel that tests for sensitivity to the four primary individual food antigens (gluten, milk, eggs, and soy) and includes a gene test for understanding your genetic predisposition to gluten sensitivity and celiac disease.

L. Lactobacillus and Bifidobacterium (Take a high-quality probiotic.)
Why It Matters: Probiotics help heal the gut, support your microbiome, unlock optimal digestion, boost weight loss, support your immune system, and promote overall health.

Today's Action Step: Start taking a high quality probiotic every day I use and recommend Strengtia (K-61) from Apex Energetics, but there are several great ones on the market. Make sure your probiotic of choice supplies at least 10 billion colony-forming units. If they're lower than that, they're not worth your money.

The Next Level: In addition to your daily probiotic supplement, make fermented foods like plain dairy-free yogurt (Silk yogurt made from almonds or SO Delicious yogurt made from coconut milk), traditionally prepared sauerkraut, kombucha, kimchi, or traditionally made pickles a regular part of your diet.

T. Time to Heal

Why It Matters: Have you ever built or remodeled a home? It always takes 40–50 percent longer than you expect. Healing the body is the same way. It didn't become dysfunctional overnight, and it's not going to heal overnight. It needs plenty of time, rest, and support to fully heal itself.

Today's Action Step: Commit to giving your body ample time to heal. Resist rushing the process or giving unrealistic expectations a foothold.

The Next Level: Write out the ultimate life you envision then go back and review this vision statement whenever you're feeling discouraged or rushed in your health journey.

H. Hydrochloric Acid (HCL)

Why It Matters: When digesting food, your stomach acid should have a pH level of 1.5–2.5. When the level of acidity is off in the stomach, all kinds of problems occur. First, if the stomach doesn't have enough HCL, food isn't broken down properly, and the possible viruses, bacteria, and parasites in our food aren't destroyed. Second, the next steps of digestion aren't triggered properly. The domino effect we talked about earlier doesn't take place. Almost no one over the age of sixty is producing enough HCL.

Today's Action Step: Start taking EnzymixPro (K99) from Apex Energetics. This HCL supporting supplement ensures your food is properly broken down and the next steps of digestion are triggered correctly.

The Next Level: Add apple cider vinegar to your diet and do your vagus nerve stimulation daily.

The ABCs TO HEALTH are a simple, easy-to-follow recipe to wellness. By following these steps, you're sending yourself squarely down the middle of the highway to health. They aren't complicated or expensive, but for fun, let's simplify these action steps even more. Pretend you're sitting across from me at my office and ask, "Dr. Bowman, what are the top three most important things I can start doing today to improve my health?"

This is my answer:

1) Get your HCL levels cranking. Having the right amount of acidity in the stomach is absolutely critical to setting up the rest of your gut for success. Order the Apex Energetics "K99" EnzymixPro today, and take it daily after every meal.

2) Stop eating gluten and casein today. They are detrimental to your health and devastating to your gut. Cut them out now, and start a detox program like the ten-week Brain and Body Detox from Apex Energetics.

3) Get out and get walking. Commit to walking for at least twenty minutes per day, four days a week. This form of exercise is easy, free, and takes minimal time, yet it stimulates your body, which in turn stimulates your brain and vagus nerve, increases your oxygen supply, and improves your mood.

Now that you've read the recipe to the highway to health, let's walk through the way every bite you take directly impacts your gut-brain connection.

CHAPTER 7

THE TEN-STORY BUILDING IN YOUR BODY

We are all here for a reason. Stop being a prisoner of our past. Become the architect of your future.

—Robin Sharma

THE TEN STORIES

Digestion is a complex process, but it doesn't have to remain a mystery. Digestion is meant to mechanically break down food (which happens in the stomach) while absorption of food products occurs in the small intestine and is assisted by the liver, gallbladder, and pancreas. We can easily understand all the steps of digestion using the analogy of a ten-story building. You can only get from the top of the building to the bottom by going through every floor, just like digestion. Every part of the process is important and sets up the next step to complete its role.

FLOOR #10: CHEWING

Digestion runs from top to bottom and in the same way, our analogy begins on floor number ten. Imagine you've just taken a big bite of an apple. This triggers the start of the digestive process, which actually begins in your mouth. Pro tip: chew your food at least twenty times to cue the enzymes needed to kick off proper digestion. Chewing is the mechanical breakdown of food, and the "muscles of mastication" are run by cranial nerve number five.

FLOOR #9: SALIVATION

Run by cranial nerves seven and nine, salivation produces saliva that contains special enzymes that start digesting your food. An enzyme called amylase breaks down starches into sugars, and an enzyme called lingual lipase begins breaking down fats.

FLOOR #8: SWALLOWING

Swallowing involves the upper esophageal sphincter and lower esophageal sphincter, which are both controlled by the vagus nerve. From this point forward, the autonomic nervous system takes over, and we no longer have conscious thought about our digestion. When things go awry at this stage, you may experience acid reflux, which happens when the lower esophageal sphincter allows acid from the stomach back up into the esophagus. Traditional doctors usually prescribe proton pump inhibiting medications like Prilosec or Nexium for this condition. Unfortunately, these drugs cause more problems down the line because they actually change the pH level of the stomach. Studies have linked the use of proton pump inhibiting medications to an eight to nine times increase in colon cancer. Signs that your lower esophageal sphincter is malfunctioning include regularly burping forty-five to fifty minutes after eating food, getting acid reflux when lying down at night, or bloating, distension, and gas.

FLOOR #7: STOMACH

Also controlled by the vagus nerve, this is where food is further broken down by the enzyme pepsin and HCL into chyme.

FLOOR #6: GALLBLADDER

Prompted by HCL production in the stomach, the gallbladder contracts and releases bile into the small intestine, which aids in breaking down fats. If you have pain in the upper right quadrant of your torso sixty to seventy-five minutes after eating, that's a sign that your gallbladder is struggling.

FLOOR #5: SMALL INTESTINE

This is where the majority of our food is digested and absorbed. The lining of the small intestine resembles a screen door (keeps the bugs out, lets the air in), and it's what protects us from the outside world that's in our food. This lining is made of tiny tight junctions that have microvilli (think little squiggles that resemble shag carpet) coming off of them. When things are working as they should, these tight junctions are so close together that only good things can pass through (e.g., amino acids, vitamins, minerals) into the portal vein that passes through our liver and ends up in our bloodstream. When leaky gut happens, those tight junctions loosen and become leaky, allowing all kinds of bad things to pass through (e.g., undigested proteins, gluten, bacteria) that should not get through the lining of the small intestine.

FLOOR #4: LIVER

The liver's job is twofold: 1) producing bile, which it sends to the gallbladder, to break down fat for digestion and 2) filtering everything that comes from our small intestine before it reaches our bloodstream. Everything we put in our mouths is filtered through our liver.

FLOOR #3: PANCREAS

The pancreas releases crucial digestive enzymes that break down proteins, sugars, fats, and starches. Your pancreas also helps your digestive system by making hormones (insulin being one of them), which are the chemical messengers that travel through your blood. If you have pain or discomfort roughly two hours after eating protein, that could be a sign your pancreas is struggling.

FLOOR #2: COLON

There are three divisions of the colon: 1) ascending, 2) transverse, and 3) descending. The main job of the colon is to absorb water from feces before it's eliminated from the body. It's also home to our microbiome.

FLOOR #1: ELIMINATION THROUGH THE RECTUM

The final step of digestion is getting rid of the remnants by ejecting them out of the rectum.

Along this path of digestion, if we have problems with any of these "stories" or phases, we always work top down to find the origin of the dysfunction. Armed with this new knowledge, here are the action steps you can take today to make sure you're on the highway to gut and brain health.

1. METABOLIC SUPPORT

The most important thing you can do is get all the equipment working on the inside. Start caring for your gut and brain health by following the ABCs to Health (see the previous chapter) and completing a ten-week brain and body detox. Why invest in the ten-week detox? It will accomplish several important metabolic goals: 1) helps with focus and attention disorders, anxiety, insomnia, and depression by detoxing your brain and gut; 2) decreases pain and inflammation by detoxing your body; 3) helps heal the gut lining which is crucial to your long-term health because seventy percent of your immune system is in your gut; 4) probably causes a fifteen to twenty pound weight loss; and 5) helps detox the liver and pancreas.

2. LAB WORK AND METABOLIC TESTING

If you're serious about healing your body, untangling the web of dysfunction, and getting on the highway to health, these tests are game changers. I recommend the following tests to create a clear, comprehensive picture of your current health:

1. Chem 77 blood test, which analyzes glucose, inflammation, anemia, liver and kidney function;
2. Enterolab A2 panel, which detects gluten and celiac genes as well as malabsorption issues;
3. Cyrex Array #2, which is the leaky gut test; and
4. Cyrex Array #5, which reveals any kind of autoimmune disorder you have brewing or that has already manifested.

If you're living with chronic health problems or you simply want to be proactive about your health and longevity, the information revealed through these tests is crucial.

3. EXERCISE CONSISTENTLY

At the risk of sounding like a broken record, I'll say it again. Commit to exercising for twenty minutes per day, at least four days per week.

If you want to go "all-out" for your health and have these tests done, call my office at 319-354-2468, and I'll either set you up with the tests or I'll recommend a doctor in your area who can administer them for you. I or a doctor I recommend can also get you started on the ten-week detox program and any other supplements you need. In the next chapter, we're going to discuss the leaky gut, break down what causes this condition, and look at ways we can solve this problem.

CHAPTER 8

LEAKY GUT

Success is a personal standard, reaching for the highest that is in us, becoming all we can be.

—Zig Ziglar

WHAT IS LEAKY GUT?

We've touched on this greatly misunderstood condition in previous chapters, but now let's take a chapter to really define leaky gut, identify its causes, and look at methods for healing it. This often misunderstood and overlooked condition is at the heart of many chronic illnesses, and if you struggle with a chronic disease, it may be one of the root causes of your web of dysfunction.

As in the ten-story building analogy, leaky gut appears in the small intestine. The number one way to test for this condition is the Cyrex Array #2 test. There are many signs and symptoms that can point to this diagnosis, but the only way to be sure is by doing this test. Leaky gut develops in the lining of the small intestine. Discovered in 2000 by Alessio Fasano and his team at the University of Maryland School of Medicine, this lining consists of tight junctions (aka the screen door) and microvilli (aka the shag carpet). The tight junctions look and act like a screen door, keeping the bad guys (bugs) out and allowing the good guys to pass through (a cool summer's breeze). When the lining of the small intestine is healthy, only amino acids (digested proteins that are the building blocks of life) and nutrients pass through this lining. Trouble arises when the tight junctures of an unhealthy gut lining loosen and allow undigested proteins to pass through, causing inflammation throughout the body. Think of the neighborhood kid throwing a baseball through the screen door of your house. Once the screen door is breached, bugs can get in your home and spread quickly.

Since the path from the small intestine to the bloodstream is the small intestine > portal vein > liver > blood stream, the liver is the body's first line of defense against these invaders. Once the bad guys get past the liver, they go into our blood-stream, traveling to every corner of our bodies and becoming a systemic problem. They tend to settle into whichever system of the body is the weakest link, which is why the symptoms of leaky gut can be vastly different from one person to the next. One person may suffer from frontal lobe issues like depression and focus and attention issues, whereas the next deals with parietal lobe problems of chronic pain, fibromyalgia. Still others experience gut issues such as gastric reflux, bloating, and con-stipation or numbness and tingling in the hands and feet. Each of these individuals is seeing every doctor under the sun, taking their meds, and continuing to suffer, and yet my patients tell me they've never heard the words "leaky gut" until they came to my office.

The body knows these undigested proteins shouldn't be traveling freely throughout the bloodstream, so it tries eliminating them from the body using one of the five organs of elimination: liver, lungs, skin, kidneys, and colon. Interestingly, rates of cancer in all of these organs of elimination are skyrocketing. Could it be that our systems are overworked, overstressed, and maxed out to the point that our God-given methods of elimination can't keep up? The rates of disease in these organs certainly point in that direction.

When a person's gut is leaky, they may experience symptoms in a variety of ways. Even though your root issue is a leaky gut, your greatest symptom may not be gut-related at all. It could be settling and manifesting elsewhere in the body. Here are the main three areas I see leaky gut symptoms appear in my patients:

1. In the body, symptoms appear as joint pain, fibromyalgia, or undiagnosed chronic pain.
2. In the brain, symptoms manifest as anxiety, depression, insomnia, focus and attention issues, or other neurodegenerative conditions.
3. In the gut, symptoms show up as IBS, gluten sensitivity or celiac disease, constipation, diarrhea, and bloating.

The effects of leaky gut should be thought of from two perspectives: short-term and long term. They show up in three main areas: the brain, body, and gut. In the brain, the short-term impact of leaky gut shows up as insomnia, depression, anxiety, and focus and concentration problems. If left untreated, the possible long-term effects can grow into serious diseases like Alzheimer's, dementia, and Parkinson's.

The short-term impact of leaky gut in the body can appear as joint pain, slight tingling in hands and feet, or fibromyalgia. Again, when left untreated, these less obvious symptoms progress into major obstacles like mobility and balance problems, needing the help of a cane or walker, and severe neuropathy. When looking at the gut, short-term effects of leaky gut appear as gas, stomach pain, bloating, distension, diarrhea, or constipation. In the long-term, these seemingly "normal" digestive issues grow into bigger problems like IBS, Crohn's, and other severe digestive illnesses. Leaky gut is a serious condition that should be treated with urgency and commitment. One of the biggest misconceptions in the medical world today is that leaky gut is a figment of holistic doctors' imaginations, not the root cause of chronic disease for millions of people around the world.

There's perhaps no area of disease where this is more misunderstood than in neurological disorders. Brain degeneration, such as Alzheimer's, typically happens in seven stages, and when you know the seven stages, you're able to pinpoint where you or your loved ones may be on the spectrum.

BRAIN DEGENERATION DOMINO EFFECT: (SEVEN STAGES OF ALZHEIMER'S)

Stage 1: Normal outward behavior.

Stage 2: Very mild cognitive changes and mental fatigue. I've seen this in patients as early as thirty years of age.

Stage 3: Mild decline. Focus, attention, and concentration issues and/or brain fog. Again, I have seen this in patients as early as thirty years of age.

Stage 4: Moderate decline. Working memory issues. Getting lost in conversation. You walk in a room and forget why you walked in the room. You can't remember where you parked your car at the mall. Usually I see this in patients in their fifth or sixth decade of life. You, your family, and even your doctor shrug it off, saying, "You're getting older, you know." Give me a break. This is not normal. It's common, but not normal.

Stage 5: Moderate to severe decline. You lose your keys, phone, remote, or coffee cup. You think others are playing tricks on you because you keep losing things. You get lost while driving. You start blaming others for all your problems.

Stage 6: Severe decline. You can't remember the name of your spouse or children. It is a very sad situation for everyone involved.

Stage 7: End stage. Unable to walk and requires significant assistance with ambulation. This stage lasts an average of 2.5 years.

Here's the point: if you are waiting for a dementia or Alzheimer's diagnosis, it probably won't happen until the fifth or sixth stage, and by then it's too late. Think of all the years and decades wasted where you could've been treating the root cause. Leaky gut is not a condition to be taken lightly. Even though the brain, body, and gut symptoms may start out mild, if left unchecked, this condition will tarnish your quality of life and create a web of health dysfunction.

With all of this talk about why we should take leaky gut seriously, it's natural to ask, "Well, where does it come from?"

Here are the three leading causes of leaky gut:

1. Prior head trauma. This could be from a car wreck twenty years ago or a sports injury in high school. Studies have shown that within six hours of head trauma, you may develop a leaky brain and a leaky gut because of the stress and shock to the brain and vagus nerve. Very few doctors will ever ask you about your past head trauma if you see them for gastrointestinal issues or brain-based symptoms, yet the science is clear: brain trauma decreases firing of the brain > decreases firing of the vagus nerve > decreases activation of tight junctions in the small intestine > creates leaky gut > bad bugs flow through portal vein > reach and pass through liver > systemic inflammation.

2. Glucose dysregulation. This issue leads to inflammation in the brain, gut, and body, causing the brain to slow down. When the brain slows down, this domino effect occurs: brain activity decreases > vagus nerve can't maintain the integrity of the tight junctions in small intestine > creates leaky gut > bad bugs get through portal vein to liver > systemic inflammation.

3. Gluten sensitivity. This leads to systemic inflammation and potential autoimmunity to brain, gut, and body tissues. Talk about a double whammy. Again, this leads to slowing down the brain > decreased function of the vagus nerve > inability to maintain tight junctions > leaky gut > portal vein > systemic inflammation.

LEAKY GUT SOLUTIONS

Healing a leaky gut is a process requiring time, consistency, and commitment. Like all chronic health problems, it didn't become dysfunctional overnight, and it's not going to heal overnight either. However, you can get on the highway to health by healing your leaky gut and supporting your gut-brain connection through the following actions:

1) Stop eating processed foods, dairy, and gluten.
2) Increase your fiber and nutrient intake by eating more natural, colorful fruits and vegetables.
3) Add high-quality probiotics and naturally prepared fermented foods to your daily diet.
4) Bonus Action Item: Take your healing to the next level by committing to a ten-week Clearvite and RepairVite Brain and Body Detox.

When you take these daily steps to change your habits and heal your leaky gut, you'll notice several results. First, if your gut is in the condition of most Americans, you'll experience a seven- to ten-day detox period. Why does this happen? Because changing your diet and eating clean essentially starves all the bad bugs in your gut, and when they starve, they begin to die. As they die off, they release waste products and toxins. This "die-off" effect may create unpleasant cramping, diarrhea, and sometimes constipation. Typically the more intense your detox phase, the more toxic your gut was in the beginning. The great news is that once your gut is cleaned out, you immediately begin reaping the rewards of your hard work and commitment. Your focus, attention, concentration, and ability to sleep soundly will improve. Your chronic aches and pains will lessen. Your attitude will likely improve, and you may lose weight. Your overall inflammation will decrease immensely, and your energy should skyrocket.

Making these lifestyle changes shouldn't be painful or miserable. Like any new habit, there will be an adjustment period. It'll take two weeks for your taste buds to adjust to your new way of eating, and you'll have to learn new ways of satisfying those sweet treat cravings, but you can do it. Instead of eating a candy bar, grab an apple. Rather than eating a slice of pie for dessert, enjoy some dairy-free yogurt topped with fresh-cut fruit. Give yourself time and grace as you learn a new way of living and eating. I promise the results you'll feel will be worth every sacrifice. Now that we've covered leaky gut and its relationship to autoimmune disorders, let's move to the next key to solving chronic health problems: controlling stomach acid.

CHAPTER 9

WHEN FOOD BECOMES YOUR ENEMY

It is never too late to be the person you might have been.

—George Eliot

WHAT IS HYPOCHLORHYDRIA?

This all-to-common condition happens when the stomach doesn't produce enough hydrochloric acid (HCL). When we're digesting food, the pH balance (level of acidity) of the stomach should be between 1.5 and 2.5. The scale of acidity ranges from zero to fourteen with zero being the absolute most acidic and fourteen being the most alkaline, or basic. When the pH level of the stomach becomes too basic, problems arise because there's not enough acid in the stomach to properly digest food. When the stomach isn't acidic enough, a cascade of negative effects occur.

First, our food isn't totally broken down, allowing undigested proteins to pass through into the small intestine. This stresses the lining of the small intestine and sets the stage for leaky gut. It also means our bodies can't break down our food products into vitamins and minerals. Second, the proper amount of HCL is needed to kill the bad bugs, parasites, and viruses that come into our systems in and on our food. Third, a shortage of HCL means other important steps of digestion which should be cued by HCL aren't activated. Steps like prompting the gallbladder to release bile or the pancreas to release essential digestive enzymes are missed because there's not enough HCL to trigger the action. The fourth negative side effect of too little HCL is a bit counterintuitive. Acid reflux is thought to happen when you have too much stomach acid, but the opposite is actually true. Most often, acid reflux is a result of too little stomach acid also known as hypochlorhydria.

When hypochlorhydria is reversed, you'll notice the following positive effects:

1) Diminished bloating, gas, and belching.

2) Protein is properly broken down into essential amino acids, the molecules that are the right size to easily pass through the lining of the small intestine. If you're curious how the breakdown of protein relates to battling depression, one of the amino acids needed to produce serotonin (the "happy" hormone that stabilizes mood and nurtures feelings of well-being) is tryptophan. If your body can't break protein down into tryptophan, it can't produce enough serotonin, which leads to anxiety and depression symptoms.

3) Your body correctly breaks down essential vitamins and minerals providing relief from malabsorption syndrome.

4) The proper amount of HCL in the stomach relieves IBS, spurs the gallbladder to work properly, and prompts the pancreas to release digestive enzymes to break down fats, proteins, and carbs.

As you can see, having the right level and amount of stomach acid is important for every stage of digestion. The good news is that we can reverse hypochlorhydria with a few simple lifestyle and diet adjustments. When we get the fundamentals of digestion right, we can sit back and let the body heal. Think of optimizing your digestion as pouring the foundation of a home. Nothing else in the home can be square, sturdy, and long lasting unless the foundation is laid correctly. The tell-tale symptoms of hypochlorhydria are:

1. Heartburn and acid reflux. This condition is actually a symptom of an environment that's not acidic enough. For example, a reduced amount of stomach acid can lead to an increase of intra-abdominal pressure (IAP), which can cause the lower esophageal sphincter to open, allowing small amounts of stomach acid to touch the esophagus and cause the familiar burning sensation experienced in gastric reflux.

2. Gallbladder discomfort. If you feel discomfort on the right side of your torso, under your rib cage, about an hour after eating, this can be a sign that your gallbladder is sluggish. Your gallbladder becomes sluggish when it's not contracting properly and releasing bile to help break down fats. This happens when there's not enough HCL to trigger the gallbladder to contract as it should.

3. Pancreas pain. If you feel pain in your upper abdomen about two hours after eating, this can be a sign your pancreas isn't producing or releasing enough digestive enzymes to break down protein and starchy foods. If your pancreas isn't producing enough enzymes, you may also notice flatulence or diarrhea after eating green, leafy vegetables.

Why does this happen? What causes someone's stomach to lack HCL? The first and most mysterious cause of hypochlorhydria is past trauma to the brain. The vagus nerve has to stimulate and activate the stomach to kick off digestion. Head trauma from many years previous can damage the brain and/or vagus nerve, slowing down communication between the brain and the gut. This dysfunction takes months or years to build up, so most people (and their doctors) don't correlate it with the digestive problems they're having today. Car wrecks, football injuries, soccer collisions, falling off a horse, a cheerleading injury, a four-wheeler wreck: the list goes on. All of these head injuries contribute to chronic health issues later in life.

The next reason hypochlorhydria develops is a rogue bacteria called *H. pylori*. This bad actor is present in the guts of 50–75 percent of the world's population, and for many, it doesn't cause a problem. Unfortunately, it can get into the stomach and wreak havoc on your health and HCL production. If it grows out of control, it drastically alters your stomach and gut function. If you have stomach or duodenal ulcers, definitely ask your doctor about being tested for *H. pylori*. The third and most common reason people don't produce enough HCL is age. Production of hydrochloric acid goes down drastically after the age of sixty.

HYPOCHLORHYDRIA SOLUTIONS

Now let's talk about methods of fixing the problem so you can get back to living your best life. The first and most important thing to rule out is an *H. pylori* infection. *H. pylori* overgrowth is serious and can lead to ulcers in your stomach. The most common treatment for *H. pylori* is antibiotics. There is a time and a place for prescription drugs, and this is one of those times. There are also nutraceuticals that manage it.

The second step is to start drinking two ounces of raw, organic apple cider vinegar every day. You can drink it straight or dilute it in water and sip on it throughout the day. This daily cocktail helps stimulate the production of HCL. The third step to reversing hypochlorhydria is taking a high-quality digestive enzyme supplement after every meal. I use and recommend EnzymixPro (K99) from Apex Energetics. EnzymixPro (K-99) not only helps maintain optimal stomach acid but also supports gallbladder, liver, and pancreatic function.

When your hypochlorhydria is reversed, you can expect your body to run a whole lot more efficiently. After you eat, you should feel nothing other than a sense of fullness. If you're having symptoms after you eat, something in the digestive tract may be malfunctioning. You shouldn't feel sleepy, tired, or sluggish, have gas, belch, or get acid reflux. Those things are common for unhealthy people but not normal. Once digestion is happening properly, our body becomes much more efficient at doing its job and healing itself.

Next comes a cascade effect of improvements in your life. In fact, you may feel so good that you surprise yourself and your loved ones. Once your gut is healed, you are less likely to experience depression, anxiety, excess fatigue, and headaches. Inflammation should go down, chronic pain should go away, and blood sugar should be regulated. Your focus, attention, and concentration should be optimized. You see, living life with these symptoms is like looking through dirty glasses. We get used to it over time, and it's not until you take those glasses off and clean them that you realize how blurry of a view you had. These aren't easy, "take a pill and fix it immediately" solutions. You need the help of a professional functional medicine doctor to guide you through this healing process. Now that we've addressed the elephant in your stomach, let's talk about the next place you can support your gut-brain connection: your microbiome.

CHAPTER 10

THE MICROBIOME

*Too many of us are not living our dreams
because we are living in our fears.*

—Les Brown

WHAT IS THE HUMAN MICROBIOME?

Discovered in the 1840s but not widely studied or talked about until the 1990s, the microbiome is the most important organ you've probably never heard about. Its role in our bodies is vital and complex. In this chapter, we're going to define the microbiome, understand where it's located and what it does, and talk about ways we can support it and help it flourish.

Our microbiome is made up of trillions of bacteria, viruses, fungi, and other microscopic living things, over a thousand species in total. These little guys are referred to as microorganisms (microbes), hence the name "microbiome." Most of the microbes in your gut live in a pocket of your large intestine called your cecum, and they are collectively called the "gut microbiome." We have ten times the number of microbes in our gut as we have cells in our body. In total, this microbiome weighs between three and five pounds, and it also communicates with our brains via the vagus nerve. The bacteria in the microbiome help digest our food (especially fiber), regulate our immune system, protect against other bacteria that cause disease, and produce vitamins. One of those is vitamin B12, which is a cofactor in DNA synthesis and aids in amino and fatty acid metabolism. Another is thiamine (vitamin B1) which helps to turn food into energy and keep the nervous system healthy. Then there's riboflavin (vitamin B2), which is important for body growth, helps in red blood cell production, and aids in the release of energy from protein. Finally, there's vitamin K, which is needed for blood coagulation and affects your weight and your brain health.

Without the gut microbiome, it would be impossible to survive. This colonization of microbes starts from the time you're born. Vaginal birth (baby picks up mom's microbes while going through the birth canal) and breastmilk are crucial for establishing a healthy microbiome. As you get older, your microbiome becomes more diversified, and higher microbiome diversity is considered good for your health.

As Healthline.com states, "The microbiome is to our gut health like breathing/oxygen is to our lungs. This is the next generation of health care. We can't live without either one."

When the microbiome is healthy and everything is functioning properly, you easily digest your food without gas, bloating, belching, diarrhea, or constipation. Your digestion is seamless and totally unnoticeable. Your mental health is also in tip-top shape. You may experience less anxiety, depression, or insomnia. You may also notice less joint pain or unexplainable fatigue. Sounds like a wonderful life, right?

We start seeing things go wrong when the microbiome isn't cared for or acknowledged. The three biggest causes of an unhealthy gut microbiome are 1) antibiotic use, 2) the standard American diet and lifestyle, and 3) hypochlorhydria. The gut microbiome is a balancing act. Fungi, yeast, and bacteria all live together in a cohesive environment, and antibiotics disrupt that ecosystem because they kill the good bugs along with the bad ones. When this happens, fungi like candida (a naturally occurring kind of yeast in the gut) grows out of control and inhibits the large intestine from doing its job. This overgrowth of yeast can grow backward through our digestive system, reaching all the way into our mouths. If you stick out your tongue and it's covered in a thin, white film, that's a sign of candida overgrowth. Often just referred to as "candida," this imbalance damages the gut's ability to digest food properly, which often leads to weight gain, anxiety, depression, and bloating.

I mentioned earlier that the largest concentration of the microbiome lives in the cecum. Next to the cecum is an important sphincter known as the ileocecal valve. This crucial valve is the gateway between the ileum (the last part of the small intestine) and the colon (the first portion of the large intestine), and its job is to allow digested food materials to pass from the small intestine into your large intestine. When this valve malfunctions, things literally "go backward," and bacteria that should be in the colon backs up into the small intestine due to ileocecal valve failure. This condition is known as small intestinal bacterial overgrowth (SIBO). It's a serious problem that can cause major bloating, distension, and discomfort.

The ileocecal valve is supposed to be a one-way valve that only lets food products pass from the small intestine to the large, so what causes it to malfunction? Vagus nerve damage, gluten exposure, inflammation, hypochlorhydria, and gastric surgery can all stress this important sphincter. Yes, the ileocecal valve is controlled by your friend and mine, the vagus nerve.

I've been in practice since 1999, and one of the most commonly overlooked areas with patients suffering from chronic health issues such as brain fog, focus problems, depression, anxiety, insomnia, chronic pain, chronic fatigue, fibromyalgia, headaches, peripheral neuropathy, and small intestinal bacterial overgrowth is the gut-brain/brain-gut axis. If you're dealing with a chronic disease, especially something like anxiety or depression, how many doctors have asked about your gut health? I'm willing to guess the answer is zero.

The gut-brain connection is so incredibly powerful and the health of all three parts—brain, gut, and vagus nerve, affects our entire bodies in ways that most traditional doctors don't acknowledge. I see things differently. Instead of looking at our bodies as many independent organs and systems, I see it as a holistic system. So when I have a patient complaining of joint pain and experiencing depression, I look at the whole human, not just the areas with symptoms. For you to have truly vibrant health, all these systems have to work together seamlessly, and the vagus nerve is the path that connects them all. If one part above fails, it's a domino effect that causes a cascade of dysfunction down through the rest of the system.

MICROBIOME SOLUTIONS

How can we support our microbiome and the trillions of organisms that comprise it? Here are four simple steps you can start taking today for a healthier gut.

1) Limit the use of antibiotics. Overuse of antibiotics is one of the most common destroyers of a healthy gut microbiome. However, please consult with your doctor before changing your medications.

2) Stop eating a standard American diet and living a standard American lifestyle.

3) Start taking a high-quality probiotic, and add fermented foods like yogurt, kombucha, kimchi, and sauerkraut to

your diet. We want to support the microbiome with additional good bacteria, and both of these methods accomplish that goal.

4)   Start doing regular vagus nerve exercises.

The most important thing I want you to take away from this chapter is that what you put in your mouth has to be absorbed and assimilated to be beneficial to your brain, body, and gut. If we continually live a lifestyle that damages our gut-brain connection, pretty soon it won't matter what we eat because our bodies won't absorb it anyway. An example of this is the name brand antacid Tums marketing a version of their product with added calcium. Tums make your stomach so basic (aka alkaline) that your body can't absorb the extra calcium anyhow. An acidic stomach is required to break down and absorb vitamins and minerals.

Like the ABCs to Health in Chapter Six, the steps to care for your gut microbiome aren't complicated or fancy, but they do require commitment and consistency. When we get the fundamentals of health right, our gut-brain connection can thrive and our bodies can heal. Can you see a future where your chronic health problems don't hold you back from living the life you desire? I can! In the next chapter, we're going to talk about a plan to accomplish exactly that kind of vision.

CHAPTER 11

THE STANDARD BOWMAN DIET

*When you know what you want,
and you want it bad enough,
you'll find a way to get it.*

—Jim Rohn

YOUR PLAN MOVING FORWARD

Now that you understand the gut-brain connection and how it impacts nearly every area of your health, it's time to make a plan of action. You can build the optimal lifestyle and develop habits that will support and promote a healthy gut-brain connection, and these changes can completely change your life. Yes, change is hard. Commitment and discipline are hard. Do you know what else is hard? Waking up in pain every day. Struggling with crippling depression and anxiety. Being overweight. Those things are hard too. It's time to "choose your hard." One path offers hope. What is the other offering you? Declining health? A lackluster future? Choose your hard.

PRINCIPLES OF THE PLAN

1. You don't have to like every change, but you do need to love the results. You may not enjoy every step of this process, but again, what's your alternative? Life at an 8–10 pain level? Is that really the quality of life you're looking for?

2. Define your goal. What is your goal? Be honest with yourself, and take some time to write down where you are now and where you want to go. If this plan could get you as close to a pain level of 1 as possible, would you do it? Would you make those changes to live a vibrant, healthy life again?

3. Embrace this principle: if you create a positive mindset, take positive actions, and maintain positive habits, you will likely reap positive results. If you create a negative mindset, take negative actions and maintain bad habits, you'll likely reap bad results. We live in a sowing and reaping world. What you put into this plan is what you'll get out of it.

Imagine someone who is financially bankrupt comes to you and asks, "What can I do to get my finances back on track?"

Hopefully you'd answer, "Stop spending more than you're earning." Being bankrupt in health is the same way. Stop making the problem worse. Get rid of the bad habits that got you in this predicament and embrace a new way of living.

What is bankrupting your health? After reading this book, you know that the standard American diet and lifestyle are huge contributing factors. You also know that unaddressed past trauma can be contributing factors too, but now you're empowered and educated. You can make these changes! Take what you've learned in this book and start applying that knowledge. Start making deposits in your health bank account.

As my final encouragement to you, if you read this whole book and only make three changes, these are the three I hope you embrace:

1) Stop eating the standard American diet. Kick the high fructose corn syrup, hydrogenated oils, excess sugar, processed carbs, and nutrient-devoid food to the curb, and never let it back in your home. Start eating whole, unprocessed fruits and vegetables. Eat real meats and healthy fats.

2) Stop living the standard American lifestyle by sitting on the couch and numbing your emotions with a screen. Start walking outside, every day if possible. Take time to breathe deeply and fill your lungs with oxygen. Allow your mind ten silent minutes to focus on positive thoughts and wander away from the stressors of day-to-day life.

3) Completely eliminate gluten and casein from your diet. They are detrimental to your long-term health.

I know these changes may seem daunting, but I am doing these things right alongside you. I'm not a rebel without a cause who wants to make your life inconvenient, boring, or difficult. My family and I have personally seen and felt the positive effects of living this way. I'm leading from the front and doing far and above what I'm asking you to do in this book. There's a reason I'm fifty years old, take zero prescription medications, and have a healthy, vibrant life.

As your friend and doctor, I implore you to take responsibility for your life and health and stop taking advice from people who have no idea what they are talking about. Set goals and write out a vision of the life you dream about. Once you have that goal, you can get through the tough moments when you don't want to execute the process. We all have days where we want to sit on the sofa and eat chips, but that's not the recipe for great health and a great life. Your legacy is too important to be wasted on the couch eating chips. You matter more than that, and as long as you're here and breathing, God isn't done with you. You have a purpose and a mission on this earth. If you want to reclaim your life from chronic disease, I'm ready to help. I'm here to help patients who want their life back, and by healing your brain, gut, and vagus nerve, you'll ultimately heal your body and reclaim your life.

PART THREE

MOVING FORWARD TODAY

CHAPTER 12

HOW EXAMS HELP YOU HEAL

WHAT IS AN EXAM?

In our clinic, every patient's journey begins with a thorough functional neurological exam. This is a head-to-toe neurological evaluation on you. We do this because we treat every single person as a unique, one-of-a-kind case. Think of the way a detective picks up the trail of a murder case that's gone cold. That's how we approach each person's tangled web of dysfunction. The exam is like cracking open that file and looking at every piece of evidence in a new light.

Many times, exams are used more as a "check off" list for doctors. They're such a rich opportunity for the doctor to gather valuable data about their patient, yet they don't bother to ask enough questions or get the right kind of data needed to really solve the patient's problems. Too often, doctors come in with preconceived notions and they don't put their hands on their patients (yes, you actually have to touch your patient to do a neurological exam).

In my experience, performing a thorough neurological exam is both an art and a science. The art aspect focuses on how to perform the exam fluidly and in a systematic way that identifies which systems are not functioning properly and are likely damaged. It's also an art form to identify and then assist the most devastated areas of the patient's brain. The science portion comes from all the neurology in classroom learning at the universities as well as textbooks. Most doctors can do the science part. It's the art part that's rare.

I use the same acronym to guide me through every single patient exam, and it's called POPQRST.

P – Primary complaint. What health issue is having the biggest negative impact on their life? Has anyone else in their family had this issue before?

O – Onset. When did the symptoms start? And is the primary complaint staying the same or getting worse?

P – Pain. What provokes the pain and what makes it better?

Q – Quality of pain. Is there burning, numbness, or tingling?

R – Radiate. Does the pain radiate out or does it stay local?

S – Severity. Rank the pain on a scale of 1–10. How bad is it?

T – Time. What time of day or night is the primary complaint worse?

During this exam, we also test the patient's oxygen levels to determine if they're anemic or not. The body can't heal unless it has the proper supply of oxygen, so this is a crucial first step. We also take their blood pressure (which gives us another hint about their oxygen levels), draw blood and perform intensive blood work, and do glucose testing. All of these tests are getting baseline measurements on the patient's seven keys to health because these keys provide the clues I use to untangle their web of dysfunction and heal their chronic health problems.

During the neurological testing portion of the exam, I use a tuning fork to test the sensitivity of their nervous system. I take the tuning fork, place it on their sternum, and allow them to feel the vibration. That vibration represents a value of 10 and serves as our reference point. Then, I do the same thing but put the tuning fork against their big toe, their thumbs and their shoulders.

Next I do a 2-point discrimination test where I make sure the radial nerve (the nerve which controls sensation in the back of the arm and forearm) is intact and functioning. Then, I test the lower extremities using a two point discrimination test. I check the L-4 saphenous nerve (controls sensation to the inside of the lower leg) and L-5 superficial peroneal nerve (controls the outside of the lower leg). I follow that test with the digit span test where I evaluate the Median nerve which controls the thumb and first and second fingers. I then check Ulnar nerve sensation to part of the ring finger and little finger. Next, I perform the digit span test on the toes via the L-5 superficial peroneal nerve which controls all sensation on the top of the feet as well as all toes (except the small toe which is controlled by the S-1 sural nerve). These tests give me a good indication of how the patient's peripheral nervous system as well as the parietal lobe, located in the back half of the brain, is functioning. Next, I test their reflexes which tells me how well their motor reflexes are responding. Human beings have 10 motor reflexes, and I test all reflexes to see how well their cerebellum, brain and spinal cord are working.

CEREBELLUM TESTS

After that, I ask them to stand up, if they can, and put their feet together and close their eyes. Next, I'll ask the patient to close their eyes and put their right foot in front of the left foot. Then, I have them switch legs. I follow that exercise up by asking them to alternately lift each leg off the ground and hold it at a 90 degree angle. If your cerebellum is functioning optimally you should be able to maintain each balance/stability test for fifteen seconds. I continue the neurological part of the exam by testing them for smell, fine motor skills, and many more factors that show me the state of their neurological health.

Finger to nose test: I ask the patient to close their eyes and try to place their little finger on the tip of their nose. Fingertip to nose tip. If they miss, they probably have a decreased functioning cerebellum on the side being tested.

It's important to approach an exam with humility and curiosity because I'm working in the field of probabilities, not absolutes. If you're aspiring to be an accountant or an engineer and seeking absolute answers, this probably is not the field for you. Practically nothing in neurology is absolute. Approaching the patient as if they're a completely new, one-of-a-kind case is the most important mental shift I make every time I prepare to do an exam.

THE FUNDAMENTALS OF AN EFFECTIVE EXAM

When a patient comes into the clinic for an exam, they'll have already filled out their paperwork and we have their blood work results on hand. I start the exam by asking them some questions. Then I move into the primary pillars of executing a great exam.

Pillar One: Where is the problem? Is it neurological, metabolic or both?

Pillar Two: How much can we stimulate the system before it fatigues?

Pillar Three: Do I think I can improve this patient's well being?

Often, the exam reveals new and insightful information that helps us "crack the case." This is why I treat every single person as a unique, one-of-a-kind case. Every person's tangled web of dysfunction is different and caused by a different combination of dysfunctional processes. The exam is how we open that cold-case file and start to uncover what's going on beneath the surface.

CHAPTER 13

OUR PROGRAM

THE PHASES OF DECLINE

The "phases of decline" refer to the stages someone struggling with chronic health problems will experience as their dysfunctional process advances. While this book is ultimately about hope and the encouragement that it is often possible to stop and reverse physical damage and disorders, you also need to take these phases of decline seriously because there is a point of no return. At this point, the body becomes so damaged that it's not possible to regenerate your health to a normal state. Let's take a look at the phases of decline for the three most common maladies I see in my clinic—brain disorders, knee pain, and neuropathy.

PHASES OF DECLINE FOR BRAIN DISORDERS

Phase One: Full Health

No symptoms expressed at all.

Phase Two: Easily Dismissable Symptoms

These are things like brain fog that just won't go away, difficulty focusing and concentrating for long periods of time, and a loss of attention to the things you normally enjoy and love. At this point, your brain cells are actually dying, yet most people won't take action, instead choosing to casually dismiss the changes. The patient usually doesn't take responsibility or action, at least not yet.

Phase Three/Four: Recognizable Symptoms

At this stage, things are beginning to progress. You may walk into a room and forget why you walked in there in the first place. Or you may call someone on the phone and forget why you called them. This is an advanced stage of brain degeneration. This is the point where the adult kids may tease their parents about having "old timers" syndrome or say things like "Mom is just losing it." At this stage, it's very important to filter who you listen to. Your healthcare provider, your kids, your friends, or your spouse may laugh it off, but it's nothing to joke about. At this phase, you must stand up and take responsibility for your health. If you know something isn't right, keep pursuing a solution until you get answers.

Phase Five: The Limitation of Matter

At this stage, the brain is degenerated to the point where the person is no longer motivated and simply doesn't have the brain ability to solve their own problems. They no longer see themselves as the problem; instead, everyone else has a problem. When someone reaches this stage, it is very hard and nearly impossible to bring them back. It's a very serious case when someone gets to this stage. It's called "limitation of matter" because at this point, the brain has degenerated so far that it's unable to regenerate and repair to its former state. I don't accept patients for care who are at this stage of degeneration.

Common Treatments For Brain Disorders

These are the common in-clinic treatments that I do for brain-based disorders.

- BrainCore Neurofeedback Program – this tool instantly and non-invasively identifies brain dysfunction. I use these results to know which areas of the brain to stimulate to help it begin functioning optimally again.
- Exercise with oxygen therapy – This is simply putting an oxygen mask on the patient and having them ride a stationary bike for 15 minutes while breathing varying levels of oxygen concentration via Adaptive Contrast Oxygen Therapy.
- Hako-Med – This powerful machine helps stimulate proper nerve function.
- At-Home Exercises – Vagal stimulation exercises, 90 day brain and body detox, and proper nutritional supplementation.

PHASES OF DECLINE FOR KNEE PAIN

I classify chronic knee pain as anything that has existed for three months or longer. Most of the people who come see me for knee pain have had it for years, if not decades, and can barely walk or get out of a chair. They often have difficulty getting out of bed or off the couch, and their life is severely impacted by their pain. One of the first things I do with every knee pain patient is take a radiograph (x-rays) of the knee. We can use regenerative medicine at the clinic, but in order for that treatment to be effective, there has to be a space between the knee joint as seen on the radiograph. The space is important because it means there is still tissue present that can be rehabilitated. If there's no space, they've reached the limitation of matter and have to be referred out for a knee replacement. I don't accept everyone that comes into the office as a patient. If I do the exam and based on their results I don't think I can help them, I refer the patient to a health professional who I think can help.

However, if the radiograph shows enough spacing in the joint, I may start with a regenerative medicine treatment plan to help them eliminate their chronic pain and regain mobility. Here are some of the solutions that have worked exceptionally well for our knee pain patients.

Common Treatments For Knee Pain

- Oxygen therapy with exercise – I talked about this treatment earlier in the book, but this is simply putting an oxygen mask on the patient and having them ride a stationary bike for twenty minutes while breathing in oxygen.
- Hako-Med – This powerful machine helps stimulate proper nerve function.
- Laser therapy – This treatment decreases inflammation and pain by dilating the capillaries to promote blood flow and encourage the healing properties to access the joint.
- Neuro Reconnect – This modality activates the two main receptors of the brain so that they fire into the cerebel-

lum, spinal cord and brain to decrease pain and increase mobility.

PHASES OF DECLINE FOR NEUROPATHY

Neuropathy patients are usually the most complicated cases because neuropathy can be caused by so many different dysfunctions. These patients often have oxygen problems, glucose problems, and their brain has deteriorated because of a lack of stimulation from their feet. Many people with neuropathy also have erectile or sexual dysfunction.

> Phase One: The feet begin tingling or experiencing a pins and needles sensation.
> Phase Two: Coldness and color changes in the toes and feet.
> Phase Three: The tingling becomes a burning pain.
> Phase Four: Loss of sensation in the legs, feet, toes.

Common Treatments For Neuropathy

- Blood sugar regulation – I work with the patient to help them balance their blood sugar so their neurological system can stabilize and begin the work of healing.
- Spinal decompression – Many patients with neuropathy have L5 damage so I use decompression therapy to relieve the pressure on that area of the spine.
- Oxygen therapy with exercise – I talked about this treatment earlier in the book, but this is simply putting an

oxygen mask on the patient and having them ride a stationary bike for twenty minutes while breathing in oxygen.

- Hako-Med on their feet – This powerful machine helps stimulate proper nerve function.
- Laser therapy – This treatment decreases inflammation and pain by dilating the capillaries to promote blood flow and encourage the healing properties to access the joint.
- Neuro Reconnect – This modality activates the two main receptors of the brain so that they fire into the cerebellum, spinal cord and brain to decrease pain and increase mobility.
- BrainCore Neurofeedback Program – this tool instantly and non-invasively identifies brain dysfunction. I use these results to know which areas of the brain to stimulate to help it start functioning optimally again.
- At-Home Exercises – Brain-Body-Gut 90 day detox and proper nutritional supplementation.

CUSTOM MADE

A truly custom, one-of-a-kind healthcare program will impact your health in a way you've never experienced before because it is created uniquely for you. I don't accept everyone for care. If someone isn't fully committed, they're too neurologically damaged, or they're too far degenerated, I'm not going to take them for care and waste their time or money. When I accept someone for care, I make them a promise that I'm on this journey with them, and we're in it to win it. I will exhaust every option I know in order to optimize their recovery. However, we both need to have realistic expectations. If their expectations are beyond what

I can give them, we need to realign. I'm always going to under promise and over deliver, and sometimes tough love requires telling people the truth that they don't want to hear.

A custom healthcare program to heal your chronic disease always comes as a result of a thorough and effective neurological examination process, and it always addresses all aspects of your metabolic and neurological health. However, the truth is that if they don't follow the program I prescribe them, they're probably not going to get the results they want. No one is going to care more about your health than you. If you don't want to be well, live vibrantly, and leave a legacy, no one is going to do it for you. I'm totally committed to the patient, but they need to be "all in" too.

CHAPTER 14

TREATING
YOU WELL

We live in an information age where facts and figures are at our fingertips. The expectation others put on us and that we often put on ourselves is to figure it out—ourselves. At the beginning of this book, I told you about growing up in the Midwest and the unspoken rules that I learned to appreciate: Work hard, use common sense, and when something breaks, figure it out and fix it. However, nowhere was I expected to do it all myself. And neither should you. There is help for people who struggle with neuropathy, autoimmune conditions, pain, indigestion, brain fog, cognitive decline, and/or chronic disease. I know this because we help people with these conditions every day!

At our clinic, there is a team and intentional process in place to ensure that you feel as comfortable, welcome, and confident as possible. We value you as a person and treat you as such. Last but not least, we aim to have fun along the way! I am not sure if I accomplish the same "party feel" as the chiropractor of my youth, but my team and I make every effort to ensure that your time with us is enjoyable and well spent.

We take pride in being intentional and removing barriers. Having a medical need is hard; finding the best provider to help with that need is also difficult. We want to make the rest of the process as smooth as possible for people. Hence, in 2006, we decided to build our spacious 4000-square-foot clinic just off Interstate 80 near Iowa City. Patients often comment how easy the drive is, how visible the signage is, how simple it is to park, and how accessible our entrance is. We figure it's the least we can do.

When you come in, you are greeted warmly by our staff. You're shown around and given time to get acquainted with the place, which hopefully helps calm any nerves you have about being in a new place. We ask you to do a respectful, but not overwhelming, amount of paperwork and then walk you through our screening process to ensure I am the right person to help you.

This screening includes a confidential consultation, a brain and body examination, neurological tests, and any necessary blood work. Throughout this process, we do all we can to understand who you are, what's important to you, and your needs, hopes, and expectations. We ask you what seems to be working and what doesn't. And we let you tell us about the journey that ultimately led you to our office. We welcome questions from you and let you share any concerns you have. We realize you might be tired, weary, and at the end of your rope by the time you make it into our office—and that is okay. You are not the first person and won't be the last to try other treatment options; we see this as a positive sign and applaud you for your efforts and for not giving up. People like you are often a great fit for our approach to health.

When the feeling is mutual, we set up an appointment for you to come back, meet with me directly to discuss everything, and identify a treatment plan–a solution–for the problems. Over the next six-to-nine months, we work together through this plan. I meet with you two-to-three times a month at first, then gradually spread the appointments out after you feel comfortable and are making progress. For your initial two-or-three appointments, I invite you to bring a loved one along. As I said earlier, people need support. There is no reason to start down this path alone if you don't have to. I am happy to lead you, but I don't want you to follow me blindly. When possible, it's beneficial to have others there to help you process the plan, understand the journey, stay on track, and support you. At our clinic, we value your support system and honor their input and opinions as though they are fellow members of your team—because they are!

Together, let's gear up, figure out what's really wrong, and figure out how to fix it. Maybe you've been told you're at an end-stage disease and there is nothing more you can do. Please don't accept that. Maybe you're scared of change and uncertain about adopting a new lifestyle. But think of it this way: change is coming one way or another. If you do nothing, your life will change by getting worse. Poor health will rob you and your loved ones of the quality of life you all deserve. There is a good chance it will rob you of your life savings, as well, as medical bills are the number-one cause of bankruptcy.

The other option incorporates what you've learned in the preceding chapters. Rather than let poor health dictate what happens next in your life, YOU spearhead change and direct your body down a healthier path. I encourage you to choose this option. Remember: starting is the hardest part, and we are here to help you with that. After that, the momentum of feeling better keeps you going!

Think about it. If you are reading this book, then clearly you are not wanting to give up or accept the status quo. You want change and are ready to be the force behind it. Combined with our knowledge and coaching, you can get started and find the momentum that leads to health. Life is short, so don't put this choice off any longer. Call and schedule an appointment with us today! You have so little to lose and so much to gain: quality of life, quality time with loved ones, the ability to travel, and more. Many patients who've made that call have won back more than their health; they've won back their life. You can too!

ABOUT THE AUTHOR

Dr. Ryan Bowman, with his wife Dr. Christine Bowman, are founders of the Bowman Clinic, parent company of Bowman Chiropractic Associates and Regenerative Therapies of the Midwest.

Drs. Bowman founded their clinic in 1999 from the first order principle that the body is self-healing, providing that the interference to healing is removed. Over time, they have built a team and facility to help their patients optimize their healing capacity in this increasingly difficult environment we live in.

Drs. Bowman both graduated from the Palmer College of Chiropractic in Davenport, IA. Dr. Christine did her undergraduate studies at Coe College in Cedar Rapids, IA, while Dr. Ryan did his undergraduate studies at the University of Kansas.

When not in the office you can find them spending time with their family, getting outdoors whenever they can. Drs. Bowman have two children, Caitlyn and Adam.

ABOUT THE COMPANY

The Bowman Clinic is the result of a 25-year-and-counting dedication to helping people achieve optimal health without the use of drugs or surgery. With chiropractors at the helm, the Bowman Clinic is uniquely positioned to apply common-sense, first-order principles to help patients optimize their recovery.

Because the Bowman Clinic offers a unique and holistic approach to solving complex health problems, the clinic routinely attracts patients routinely within a two-hour driving distance from places such as Southern Minnesota, Southern Wisconsin, Western Illinois, and Eastern Nebraska to its convenient Iowa City location. This has led to the clinic experiencing significant growth in recent years, but it also remains efficient in order to offer maximum value to patients. The Bowman Clinic operates effectively with three full-time staff plus the doctors. The growth also places a responsibility on the clinic to continue moving forward as technology advances—a responsibility that the doctors humbly accept.

Website: BowmanClinic.com
Office: 319-354-2468
Address: 2501 N Dodge, Iowa City, IA 52245

REFERENCES

Suganya, K., & Koo, B.-S. Gut-Brain Axis: Role of Gut Microbiota on Neurological Disorders and How Probiotics/ Prebiotics Beneficially Modulate Microbial and Immune Pathways to Improve Brain Functions. *International Journal of Molecular Sciences*. http://www.ncbi.nlm.nih.gov/ pmc/articles/PMC7589356/.

Breakthrough study: Gastroenterology 2009

This study identifies an increase in gluten sensitivity in the US. Blood samples were collected from 1948–1954 of 9,000 healthy young adults. The researchers found the prevalence of celiac disease in increased dramatically during the past fifty years, from 1:700 to 1:100.

Kharrazian, Datis. *Why Isn't My Brain Working?: A Revolutionary Understanding of Brain Decline and Effective Strategies to Recover Your Brain's Health.* Carlsbad, CA: Elephant Press, 2013.

Kharrazian, Datis. *Why Do I Still Have Thyroid Symptoms?: When My Lab Tests Are Normal: A Revolutionary Breakthrough in Understanding Hashimoto's Disease and Hypothyroidism.* Carlsbad (CA): Elephant Press, 2010.